FROM TROUBLE AT SCHOOL TO CONFLICTS AT HOME: IF YOUR CHILD IS STUCK IN A CYCLE OF FRUSTRATION, HE OR SHE MAY BE SUFFERING FROM AD/HD

Often completely overlooked or confused with many other problems such as learning disabilities, Attention Deficit/ Hyperactivity Disorder is a biological disease that affects about three million American children and causes inappropriate behavior, poor school performance, and isolation from family and peers. But AD/HD can be treated in children of all ages throughout every stage of their lives. Now thoroughly revised and updated with the latest medical findings, this comprehensive and easy-to-understand guide offers a home-based program for helping kids with this condition. Learn how to:

- Spot the symptoms of this affliction in all students from preschool to college
- Get your child tested for AD/HD—and eliminate other possible causes of unusual behavior
- Become your child's advocate at school and even among his or her friends
- Ease your child's inner frustration and help maintain his or her self-esteem
- Develop strategies for success in the classroom
- Separate the myths from the facts about AD/HD medication, including stimulants and anti-depressants

    . . . and much more.

■   ■   ■

A crucial book for parents, AD/HD: HELPING YOUR CHILD is also an invaluable resource for teachers, daycare providers, and all professionals working with children.

AD/HD
Helping Your Child

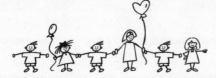

A COMPREHENSIVE PROGRAM TO TREAT ATTENTION DEFICIT/HYPERACTIVITY DISORDERS AT HOME AND IN SCHOOL

WARREN UMANSKY, Ph.D.
and **BARBARA STEINBERG SMALLEY**

WARNER BOOKS

AN AOL TIME WARNER COMPANY

This book is not intended as a substitute for medical advice of
physicians. The reader should regularly consult a physician in all
matters relating to his or her health, and particularly in respect of
any symptoms that may require diagnosis or medical attention.

Copyright © 2003 by Warren Umansky, Ph.D., and
Barbara Steinberg Smalley

All rights reserved.

Warner Books, Inc., 1271 Avenue of the Americas,
New York, NY 10020

Visit our Web site at www.twbookmark.com

An AOL Time Warner Company

Printed in the United States of America

First Printing: July 2003

10   9   8   7   6   5   4   3   2   1

Library of Congress Cataloging-in-Publication Data
Umansky, Warren.
    AD/ HD : helping your child : a comprehensive program to
treat attention deficit/hyperactivity disorders at home and in
school / Warren Umansky and Barbara Steinberg Smalley.—
[2nd ed.].
        p. cm.
    Previously published under the title: ADD : helping your
child.
    Includes bibliographical references and index.
    ISBN 0-446-67973-9
    1. Attention-deficit hyperactivity disorder. 2. Attention-
deficit-disordered children. I. Smalley, Barbara Steinberg.
II. Umansky, Warren. ADD. III. Title.

RJ506.H9 U46 2003
618.92'8589—dc21

                                            2002027447

Cover design by Brigid Pearson
Book design and text composition by Stratford Publishing Services

*We dedicate this book with deep appreciation
to the children, parents, and teachers who have
taught us so much, and to our families, who have
provided love and support during our endeavors.*

—WARREN UMANSKY, PH.D.
—BARBARA STEINBERG SMALLEY

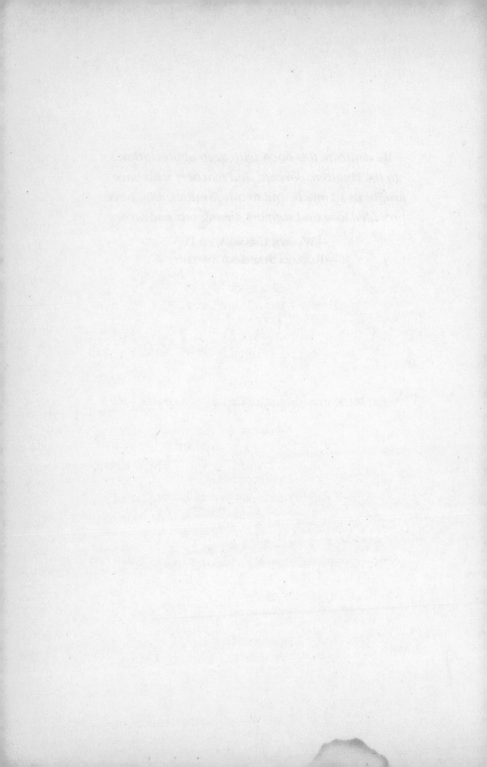

CONTENTS

Contents

INTRODUCTION

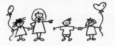

AD/HD: SEARCHING FOR ANSWERS

Attention Deficit/Hyperactivity Disorder (AD/HD) affects about three million school-age children, causing its young victims to be inattentive, impulsive, easily distracted, and—in many instances—hyperactive. This disorder often looks different in boys than it does in girls. For example, boys tend to show a higher incidence of hyperactivity, inattention, impulsiveness, and externalizing problems, such as conduct disorders. Girls with AD/HD, on the other hand, tend to have greater intellectual impairment and internalizing problems, such as depression.

While once considered a disorder that children outgrew during the teenage years—as hyperactivity does tend to decrease with age—it is now clear that many of the symptoms of AD/HD continue into adulthood.

Undiagnosed and untreated, AD/HD wreaks havoc on a youngster's sense of self-esteem and interferes with his or her abilities to perform well at school, to make friends, and to get along with siblings and parents. After all, children with AD/HD find themselves repeatedly reprimanded for doing things they can neither understand nor control. Caregivers and teachers may mistake such children's behavior and dismiss them as disruptive and uncooperative troublemakers.

Parents of children with AD/HD often hold lofty expectations for their youngsters—expectations that are shattered by a child whose behavior they cannot seem to control. AD/HD can also zap the joy out of raising children, leaving parents of young victims feeling humiliated, helpless, and wondering, "Where did we go wrong?"

Its roots are mysterious, embedded in the structures and chemicals of the brain. Treatments remain controversial. Despite the fact that it is one of the most prevalent childhood disorders, AD/HD remains one of America's most misunderstood challenges and has been the focus of thousands of scientific studies, as well as a hot topic for magazines, newspapers, and talk shows.

What Can I Do?

Any household with children is destined to be chaotic, but one with a child who has AD/HD can be particularly tumultuous.

In this book, you will learn a number of strategies to help your child and to help your child help himself. You will master new and effective ways to deal with the difficult behavior that is characteristic of children with AD/HD. You will also learn how to deal with your needs as the parent of a child with this disorder.

Maybe your child attends school or a daycare center during the day, leaving you limited opportunities to spend quality time with her. Or maybe you stay at home with your preschooler and have increased contact with him. Regardless of your situation, the underlying philosophy of this book is: *However many or few hours you spend with your child, these times should be pleasant and productive, not marked by conflict and crisis.* Childhood should be a time of growth, learning, enjoyment, and success. This book will help you find out what it takes as a special parent or caregiver to make this happen with the least amount of stress.

Granted, parenting is by nature a job filled with highs and lows. But you deserve to get satisfaction from your role, and the information and strategies in this book will show you how. Of course, no text can offer guarantees, but if you commit yourself to reading this book and following the recommendations consistently, you should experience many dramatic family changes. You will feel less frustration and anger when interacting with your child. And your child will enjoy greater success in school, social, and recreational activities—which, in turn, should enhance his self-image.

Finally, the way your entire family functions will change for the better. There will be less yelling, fewer threats made, a significant decrease in out-of-control emotional outbursts, and—best of all—greater pleasure in your role as a parent.

Much of this book will be helpful as you interact with physicians, mental health professionals, and school personnel. Some parts will be helpful to teachers, daycare personnel, and school administrators. Chapter Seven, for example, is filled with strategies that can be used in the schools. Other parts will give professionals a better understanding of the problem of AD/HD from the perspective of the child and the parents. Being familiar with these materials will allow parents and professionals to be on the same wavelength when they communicate about the needs of a particular child.

A Comprehensive Guide

When the first edition of this book was published, the thirst for information on AD/HD was profound. The complex issues surrounding this disorder were bewildering to many parents, teachers, and other caregivers. Today, much more is known about AD/HD; nevertheless, the problems still reach into the school, the community, and the family, as well as deep within the child's sense of accomplishment and self-esteem. They encompass academics, social skills, recreation, and career skills. For this reason, we have tried to fashion this book to be comprehensive yet easy to read.

Keep reading to discover the latest research on the causes and effects of AD/HD. Get information on the steps involved in assuring a proper diagnosis of this disorder for your child and how to decide if medication is the answer. Learn how to work with caregivers, teachers, and the school system to guarantee that your child with AD/HD gets the care he deserves and needs. Finally, master tried-and-true behavior management approaches that will not only minimize the stresses of raising a special-needs child, but help your child succeed and be the best he can be.

AD/HD: Helping Your Child

How I feel

*When I'm in class I don't
answer anything unless I'm
called on sometimes not
even then. I feel like it's just
an ordinary day like the rest.
It's like I'm never going to
remember anything at all, never.
I feel worthless, useless,
like I'm stupid as heck
and I don't know anything.
I feel like nothing.
I FEEL
BLANK*

*That
is
what
I
feel.*

—J.L.M., *twelve*

1

AD/HD: What It Is and Isn't

Robert, a third-grader, walks to school most days. His school is no more than a five-minute trek from home, yet even when Robert leaves on time, he is often thirty minutes late.

His classmates don't like Robert very much. They say he's bossy and claim he's always picking on them. Robert has problems in the classroom as well. He spends the majority of his time under or near his desk rather than sitting down and working. His handwriting is sloppy, his work is messy, and his assignments are frequently left unfinished. He's constantly losing things and can't seem to keep up with the class when they are reading aloud. And rarely does he have the right materials out to complete a given task.

At home, Robert is equally disorganized. His parents say he is extremely messy and has to be re-peatedly reminded to complete simple chores. In the

neighborhood, Robert has few friends his own age.
When he plays with them, a fight typically ensues over
sharing, hurt feelings, and so forth. Consequently,
Robert plays mostly with children who are older or
younger than he is.

Robert was recently diagnosed as having Attention Deficit/ Hyperactivity Disorder (AD/HD)—and he's far from alone. AD/HD is thought to affect some 3 percent to 5 percent of today's school-age children in the United States. And while this disorder seems to have emerged from nowhere to become a near epidemic over the last decade, it's hardly new.

In fact, AD/HD has been recognized since the early 1900s, and is one of the most widely researched of all childhood disorders. Over the years, however—and to reflect researchers' growing advances in concept and theory about this disorder— AD/HD has assumed many aliases.

In the 1930s, for example, children who exhibited AD/HD-like symptoms were described as having "Minimal Brain Damage." In the 1960s, that label changed to "Minimal Brain Dysfunction" and was considered relatively rare. By the 1970s, however, it was called "Hyperkinesis," and up to two hundred thousand children were thought to have the disorder.

In the late 1980s, the term Attention Deficit Disorders (ADD) was coined, and affected children were categorized as having ADD with or without hyperactivity. The current name, Attention Deficit/Hyperactivity Disorder—or AD/HD—was first used in 1994.

What Is AD/HD?

The American Psychiatric Association redefined AD/HD in 1994 to describe three subtypes:

1. **AD/HD Predominantly Inattentive.** Jill, eleven, fits this category. Though bright and intelligent, she has trouble paying attention to details, and, as a result, tends to make careless mistakes on classwork and homework. Her teachers often reprimand Jill for gazing out the window instead of listening to directions. But Jill can't help it. A chirping bird outside distracts her from the math problem in front of her.

2. **AD/HD Predominantly Hyperactive-Impulsive.** Eight-year-old Sam falls into this subtype. He's always tapping his pencil, squirming in his seat, or otherwise fidgeting in class. His teachers often send notes home saying, "Sam can't stay seated or quiet and often blurts out answers instead of waiting to be called on." At home, when friends come over, Sam has trouble waiting his turn while playing games, and he's constantly interrupting his mom when she's on the phone.

3. **AD/HD Combined Type.** A child who falls into this category is inattentive as well as hyperactive and impulsive—like Robert, whom you read about earlier. One of the reasons Robert is often late for school—even when he leaves on time—is that he might spot a frog along the way and decide to chase it for a while. Once he is in school, his teacher calls out Robert's name several times a day because he is often under or near his desk rather than sitting down working. Robert rarely finishes his assignments in the classroom, because he can't seem to pay attention long enough to complete them. And when his class is reading aloud, he has trouble keeping up with them, because his mind wanders. At home, his parents say Robert is a whirlwind. He rarely sits still, even when eating. His parents must also repeatedly remind him to do his chores and stay focused on his homework.

People used to think that AD/HD was the result of some type of brain damage, but scientists now know that's not true. Granted, the exact causes of this disorder remain a mystery; nevertheless, cutting-edge research using computerized imaging technology and other sophisticated diagnostic tools is revealing fascinating clues to why some youngsters' brains have a propensity to AD/HD, while others do not.

Scientific evidence suggests that the level of neurological activity is quite different in certain parts of the brain in individuals with AD/HD compared to those who do not have the disorder. Differences have also been found in the size of various parts of the brain. Furthermore, at least in some cases of AD/HD, these central nervous system differences appear to have a hereditary component. We will talk more about the causes of AD/HD in Chapter Three.

Some researchers have described AD/HD as an inhibition disorder. That is, children are unable to put the brakes on useless movements, can't control their distractibility and inattention, and can't overcome their tendency to daydream. It is this inhibition theory that puts AD/HD in a family with certain other disorders, such as depression, obsessive-compulsive disorder, and tics.

What It's Not

AD/HD is a biological, *not* an emotional disorder, though it can cause its victims to experience emotional problems at home, in school, and in social settings. Neither is AD/HD a learning disability, although many children with AD/HD also have learning disabilities. Nor is AD/HD caused by poor parenting or inadequate teachers, although a disorganized home life and school environment can make its symptoms worse.

Some suspect diet as the culprit, but extensive research offers proof positive that too much sugar, aspartame (brand name: NutraSweet), food additives, food coloring, and food allergies do not cause AD/HD, either. Nor does watching too much television or playing too many computer or video games, although these may reflect an environment that lacks good supervision and may nurture the development of AD/HD-like characteristics in a child.

What is true is that many children with AD/HD also suffer from other conditions, including depression, anxiety, enuresis (bedwetting), and tics. And for the frustrated parent and the unhappy child, sorting out which symptoms are biologically based, which are learned behavior, which are controllable or not controllable, and which are severe enough to interfere with the child's success presents a significant dilemma.

Of course, not all youngsters who misbehave, who have trouble paying attention in school, or who have difficulty making friends have AD/HD. In fact, a host of physical, emotional, and situational problems can masquerade as AD/HD. Which is why it's imperative that a child be properly diagnosed before being treated.

Diagnosis

With no virus or bacteria to look for, no X-rays to take or blood tests to administer, how is a diagnosis for AD/HD made? Usually it involves input from a team of professionals—and from the child's parents.

First, a medical doctor performs a thorough physical exam—which often includes neurological tests—to rule out any physical causes (such as vision problems or hearing loss) for the difficulties a child is experiencing. Many physical and medical problems, such as thyroid dysfunction, may cause behavior that mimics AD/HD. (See Chapter Two for other maladies that can masquerade as AD/HD.)

Once physical causes are ruled out, a psychologist may be consulted. She may begin by taking a comprehensive history from the child's parents and consulting with the child's teachers. In addition to asking questions about a child's level of achievement, as well as social and emotional functioning, the psychologist looks for signs of family crises (death, job loss, divorce, a recent move) that can trigger behavior problems that can be mistaken for AD/HD.

Gathering input from teachers and other caregivers is equally essential, as symptoms that appear only at school or at home may indicate that the problem is not AD/HD, but something related to a specific setting.

Classroom and home behavior is most often evaluated using checklists such as the ones shown on pages 7 and 8. These checklists allow professionals to get a better idea of a child's typical behavior—particularly behavior that may not be obvious from observation. Two different checklists are presented. One lists problem behavior while the second states positive behavior. There are many commonly used checklists for parents and teachers that incorporate one or both of these formats.

Naturally, documenting a child's behavior in different settings is an important part of the diagnostic process. In fact, for a correct diagnosis to be made, a child must exhibit symptoms in at least two different settings. Thus, the psychologist will frequently observe a child at school as part of the data-gathering process.

So, what does the psychologist look for in the school setting? A number of characteristics that can support a diagnosis of AD/HD, as well as ideas to help the child improve his or her performance in the classroom. For example, the psychologist might note how a child's seat placement contributes to distractions and how it affects his ability to copy material from the chalkboard or get assistance from another child or the teaching staff. The psychologist will likely observe how much time the child spends paying attention to assigned work versus the amount of time spent daydreaming or working on other, unassigned tasks. She might observe how the child gets along

BEHAVIOR CHECKLIST FOR PARENTS

Child's Name _____ Age _____ Sex _____

Completed by: mother _____ father _____ other _____

Behavior	Not at All	Just a Little	Pretty Much	Very Much
1. Runs or climbs excessively				
2. Has trouble staying seated for meals or homework				
3. Fidgets excessively				
4. Doesn't finish work or tasks				
5. Doesn't work independently				
6. Doesn't seem to listen				
7. Easily distracted				
8. Acts before thinking				
9. Interrupts often				
10. Is bossy or picks on other children				
11. Plays loudly				
12. Has trouble getting along with peers				
13. Shows poor self-esteem				
14. Is disorganized				
15. Loses things needed for tasks				
16. Forgetful about school assignments and tasks				
17. Makes careless mistakes				
18. Has difficulty following directions				
19. Has a hard time waiting for a turn				
20. Takes an excessive amount of time to complete homework				

Behavior Checklist for Teachers

Child's Name _____ Age _____ Sex _____

Completed by: _____

Behavior	Not at All	Just a Little	Pretty Much	Very Much
1. Completes seat work				
2. Pays attention				
3. Follows directions well				
4. Completes work				
5. Stays on task				
6. Is organized				
7. Thinks before acting				
8. Waits to be called on to respond				
9. Gets along with peers				
10. Awaits turn in games and groups				
11. Stays seated, as required				
12. Sits still				
13. Participates well in group activities				
14. Controls emotions well				
15. Works carefully				

with his peers, as well as the types of children he gets along with best—or worst.

The psychologist will likely monitor how successful the child is at paying attention to and completing independent work, and compare that to his performance in class discussions or in small groups. She will also note the frequency and intensity of the child's problem behavior—and how the teacher responds to the child.

The problem is that a child with AD/HD may show different behavior in different settings, at different times of day, with different people, and when different levels of challenge are presented. Therefore, relying on the report of one observer or formulating an impression of a child from an isolated observation may offer only a narrow view of the child's problem. For a diagnosis to be accurate, it is important to compare and contrast a child's performance under a number of conditions and to analyze observations from various individuals. For this reason, the psychologist may observe a child several times, on different days.

Can the diagnostic process move forward without the input of a psychologist? Yes, it can. But some professional must take the lead in gathering information and documentation to help the physician make a diagnosis and to help parents and teachers respond to the child's needs. The parents' professional partner may be a private or school psychologist, another mental health professional, a supportive teacher or school administrator, or even a friend who has traveled the same path.

When evaluating a child for AD/HD, professionals rely on a profile of characteristics that tend to differentiate children who might have AD/HD from those who do not. This profile is then compared with a list of criteria to make an official diagnosis.

Where do these criteria come from? They are listed in a manual that is published and revised periodically by the American Psychiatric Association. Professionals use this manual to diagnose specific psychiatric and psychological diseases and disorders, and in its most recent edition—*Diagnostic and Statistical Manual—IV (DSM-IV)*—the three types of AD/HD we discussed earlier are listed.

Defining AD/HD

Here are details of the three subtypes of AD/HD:

AD/HD Predominantly Inattentive

A diagnosis of this subtype of AD/HD requires that at least six of the following symptoms have been present for at least six months; they must interfere with normal functioning in social, academic, and occupational skills; they must be present in at least two different settings; and they must be inconsistent with the child's developmental level:

1. Often fails to give close attention to details or makes careless mistakes in school work, work, or other activities.
2. Often has difficulty sustaining attention in tasks or play activities.
3. Often does not seem to listen to what is being said to him or her.
4. Often does not follow through on instructions and fails to finish school work, chores, or duties in the workplace (not due to oppositional behavior or failure to understand directions).
5. Often has difficulty organizing tasks and activities.
6. Often avoids, expresses reluctance about, or has difficulty engaging in tasks that require sustained mental effort, such as school work or homework.
7. Often loses things necessary for tasks or activities (such as school assignments, pencils, books, tools, or toys).
8. Is often easily distracted by extraneous stimuli.
9. Often forgetful in daily activities.

AD/HD Predominantly Hyperactive-Impulsive

What was once called ADD with hyperactivity has been re-named AD/HD predominantly hyperactive-impulsive type. For a diagnosis to be made of this condition, at least some of the following symptoms must have been present before seven years of age; at least six of the symptoms must have been present for at least six months; they must interfere with normal functioning in academic, social, and academic skills; they must appear in two or more settings; and they must be inconsistent with the child's developmental level:

Hyperactivity

1. Often fidgets with hands or feet or squirms in seat.
2. Leaves seat in classroom or in other situations in which remaining seated is expected.
3. Often runs about or climbs excessively in situations where it is inappropriate (in adolescents or adults, may be limited to subjective feelings of restlessness).
4. Often has difficulty playing or engaging in leisure activities quietly.
5. Is always "on the go" or acts as if "driven by a motor."
6. Often talks excessively.

Impulsivity

7. Often blurts out answers to questions before the questions have been completed.
8. Often has difficulty waiting in lines or awaiting turn in games or group situations.
9. Often interrupts or intrudes on others (for example, butts into others' conversations or games).

AD/HD Combined Type

Diagnosing this mixed subtype of AD/HD requires that a child meet the criteria for both inattentive and hyperactive-impulsive subtypes. Moreover, at least some of the symptoms must have been present before seven years of age; they must appear in at least two different settings (at school, at home, in recreational or social settings); they must clearly impair social and academic functioning; and they must not be due to other specified developmental or psychiatric disorders.

If you are a parent, it is important that you be well-prepared in providing documentation of your child's behavior, that you be able to describe his behavior and performance in various situations, and that you consider other factors that may be causing your child to perform as he does. Professionals will use the symptoms listed above—together with other information from physical exams and reports from teachers and observed behavior—to determine if your child has AD/HD.

What's Normal, What's Not

All children are overly active some of the time. Many also have short attention spans and may act without thinking. Several factors, however, distinguish youngsters with AD/HD from those who do not have this problem.

First, it's true that many of these behavior patterns are developmental in nature. In other words, they appear in children at certain ages, but youngsters typically outgrow them. In children with AD/HD, however, many such behavior patterns persist. These youngsters either do not outgrow the behavior or the behavior disappears for a while, then returns.

Second, children with AD/HD often exhibit more such behavior than do children without the disorder. During a typical child's early years, for example, the majority of parents deal with a few of these behavior patterns. But parents of children with AD/HD deal with far more such behavior and for a much longer period of time.

Finally, parents can usually control a majority of undesirable behavior in children who do not have AD/HD by using good behavior management strategies. Youngsters with AD/HD, however, tend not to respond to most behavior management strategies or show great inconsistency in their response. A harsh reprimand, time-out, or restriction, for example, may be enough for most children to be convinced to straighten up. But these approaches are not likely to have long-lasting effects on a child with AD/HD.

Describing the Child with AD/HD

Children with AD/HD are not all the same. They may exhibit some characteristics frequently and others less frequently or not at all. Yet, having a clearer understanding of which behavior may be a consequence of AD/HD may help parents to better understand their child and to be less frustrated by their behavior. In a slight departure from the list of specific symptoms presented earlier, consider these descriptions, which characterize the kinds of behavior one most often sees in children with AD/HD:

Fidgets, Squirms, or Seems Restless

Children with AD/HD are often described as "always on the move." In the classroom, they are the toe tappers or the ones who are constantly fiddling with other objects on or in their desks. They may chew on their collar or gnaw pencils. At home, during mealtime, they may toy with their silverware or food. Children with AD/HD also often demonstrate new and creative ways of sitting in a chair: on their legs, with legs propped up on a desk or table, or half-standing and half-sitting.

Has Difficulty Remaining Seated

Teachers report that children with AD/HD are frequently out of their seats for a variety of reasons. They need a drink of water. They need to sharpen a pencil. They need to go to the bathroom. In fact, teachers agree that it's not unusual to find a child with AD/HD wandering around the classroom for no apparent reason.

At home, a youngster with AD/HD usually eats on the go because he has a difficult time remaining seated for an entire meal. Homework time also suffers, because the child is unable to sit still long enough to complete his assignments. And when it comes to enjoying activities that require participants to sit for any length of time—such as concerts, lectures, and church or synagogue services—parents often resign themselves to the fact that they cannot take their child along. If they do, they spend excessive amounts of time reminding him to remain seated and stay quiet.

Is Easily Distracted

Children with AD/HD lose their concentration very easily if there are sounds or movements around them. Consequently, in school they have difficulty focusing on independent seatwork if, for example, a reading group nearby is making noise, the classroom gerbil is exercising, or a child sitting next to them is wearing a watch with a loud ticking noise. That's because many youngsters with AD/HD are simply unable to disregard distractions like these.

Homework becomes a chore, as well, when the television or stereo is on in a nearby room, or when people are coming and going near the homework area. Oddly enough, however, children with AD/HD may appear freer from distraction when playing video games or watching television. This is likely due to the multisensory nature (sound, color, and constant action) of these activities. Consequently the ability to pay attention to these activities is not sufficient to rule out a diagnosis of AD/HD.

Has Difficulty Waiting His Turn

Many children with AD/HD can't wait in line as well as other youngsters of the same age. Some may try to force their way to the front of the line. Others fidget or constantly touch other children or things while waiting their turn, or they may gyrate or dance around in line.

Blurts Out Answers

Children with AD/HD would make ideal quiz show contestants, and they may excel at classroom drills where quick answers are rewarded. But in a structured classroom setting, these children often stand out as being impatient and uncooperative. Unable to muster the self-discipline needed to hold back an answer until they are called upon, children with AD/HD will call out an answer as soon as they think they know it.

Moreover, in some instances, their comments may be totally unrelated to the specific class activity or discussion. This probably occurs because of the associations the child makes in response to a question. For example, the question, "What is the capital of Montana?" may get the child thinking of the family trip to Montana last year, the plane landing in Helena (the capital), their horseback riding excursion at Yellowstone, and the park ranger they stopped to talk to. When the child answers, "the park ranger," there is no way for the teacher to know that the child's reply springs from having the answer, though her thoughts have speeded right past the appropriate response.

Has Difficulty Following Directions

Children with AD/HD usually fare better when dealing with a single set of instructions. In fact, many become totally lost when they are given several instructions at one time. Say a parent tells a child to put on her pajamas, brush her teeth, and come back for a "goodnight kiss." Five minutes later, the child is wandering around aimlessly or engaged in her room playing with her CD player, not having even begun to do what she was told. The same pattern occurs in school. When students are given numerous directions for several worksheets at a time, the child with AD/HD may either remember instructions for the first worksheet but not remember others, or remember instructions for the last worksheet. Consequently, these children frequently appear to be out of touch with what is going on in the classroom. They also have difficulty remembering what they are supposed to do for homework or which books to take home. Even if they write down assignments, the information may often be garbled or wrong.

Has Difficulty Sustaining Attention

A classic sign of AD/HD is the number of incomplete papers the child brings home from school. Children with AD/HD have difficulty completing assignments, and the appearance of their papers is usually a good indicator of the disorder. They may complete the first few problems on a page, but the remainder of the page is blank. Or their papers will look as if they rushed through the work in an attempt to get everything finished without regard to quality or correctness.

On the flip side, some children with AD/HD are so meticulous that they may do their work over and over until it is perfect. But this extra time devoted to perfection often prevents them from completing other important tasks on their to-do list.

Shifts from One Uncompleted Task to Another

Parents of youngsters with AD/HD often describe their children as having difficulty playing by themselves or as moving from one play activity to another without devoting much attention to any of them. Teachers agree. They describe students with AD/HD as very impulsive in learning centers and as likely to discontinue working at a project before its completion. Furthermore, these children often leave remnants of their activities around their desk, the classroom, or the house.

Plays Loudly

Even when warned to calm down, children with AD/HD have a tough time maintaining a quiet state. They are also easily aroused by other children. As a rule of thumb, the louder and busier an environment is, the louder and busier the child will be. In fact, many parents with just one child who live in a relatively quiet home often have a difficult time believing that their child with AD/HD is as busy and loud in the classroom as the teacher says he is. But after further probing, these parents usually come up with similar descriptions of how their child typically behaves with them outside the home, such as at restaurants or at the mall.

Talks Excessively

A child with AD/HD is often described as being very talkative and asking questions that are repetitive or that make little sense, "Like an out-of-control tape recorder that is locked on playback at a faster speed than normal," according to one parent. Some parents may be quick to defend such behavior: "She's perky, just like her mom," or, "He's all boy." But when it interferes with a child's success and is combined with other symptoms of AD/HD, it is reason for concern and action.

Interrupts or Intrudes on Others

Parents often describe their children with AD/HD as interrupting them constantly when they are on the telephone or when they are talking to their spouses or friends. Efforts to stop this annoying behavior are generally futile, they say—to the point that parent-child shouting matches frequently ensue. Moreover, because of this tendency not only to interfere with what others are saying but also to try to impose their will on others, children with AD/HD are often unpopular in groups.

Does Not Seem to Listen

Because children with AD/HD have trouble focusing visually and sustaining visual attention on an individual or an activity, people often assume that the child is not listening. On the contrary, many youngsters with AD/HD are still able to comprehend what is going on around them. In fact, teachers and parents are often surprised that the child is able to answer questions or repeat what has been said to him. Children with severe AD/HD, however, may not absorb what is said. In addition, many children with AD/HD may have a limited working memory, so that they cannot retain verbal directions long enough to carry them all out.

Loses or Forgets Things

Children with more severe cases of AD/HD often are so poorly organized that they never seem to know where papers, pencils, articles of clothing, or other belongings were left. They often come home without the books they need for homework, for example, or may not be able to find a shoe they just had in their hand! Nor is it unusual for them to forget to relay important written or verbal messages to their parents from their teachers—or vice versa—or to spend hours doing their homework, then lose their papers before school the next day or forget to turn them in.

Engages in Physically Dangerous Activities

Because youngsters with AD/HD tend to be impulsive, they often act before thinking. For instance, they might run out into a street after a ball without looking, jump from heights without considering potential danger, or ride a bicycle at breakneck speed without considering what is in front of them.

More Clues and Characteristics

Parents and teachers report other behavioral patterns they see at home, in school, and in the community:

Works Better One-on-One Than Independently or in Large Groups

If your child has AD/HD, you may find that homework goes much more quickly if you sit with him while he does it. Left alone to complete his homework—or classwork—a child with this disorder will more than likely be up and down, fidget, daydream, stare out the window, and not finish the work. Even sitting with your child may require constant redirection and hours of dealing with inefficient work skills. However, the fact that your child *can* do the work if you sit with him indicates his ability to master the material.

Plays Better with Older or Younger Than with Same-Age Children

Parents of children with AD/HD often worry about their child playing almost exclusively with much younger or much older children. Actually, there's a good reason why this happens. Youngsters with AD/HD are often bossy or pick on other children and, while they may get away with bossing around younger children, same-age peers won't put up with such a demanding playmate. Older children also tend to be more tolerant of this type of behavior, or the child with AD/HD may control his behavior better among older children for fear of being rejected and losing the status of being able to play with them. In any case, the child is likely to be alienated from his peers and to have more relationships with younger and older children.

A child with AD/HD may also play successfully with just one child. In group situations, however, conflicts are likely to occur. That's because in most social situations, children with

AD/HD have difficulty reading social cues. They simply don't recognize when others are sending nonverbal messages that say, "You're coming on too strong," or, "Back off."

Has Difficulty Copying Words from the Chalkboard or Book to Paper

The process of transferring information requires looking, retaining in working memory what was seen, then unloading that information onto paper. This can be a difficult process for children with AD/HD, since fleeting attention limits the amount of information that can be stored in memory from a single glance. Even when information is stored, it may be done in a faulty manner, or there may be errors (spelling mistakes, reversing information, adding or deleting information) in transferring the information from memory to paper. For youngsters with AD/HD, transferring information accurately requires many more glances at the source material, but these children are likely to tire of this quickly and may very well just write down what they *think* they saw.

Knows Material Well While Studying, Then Performs Poorly on a Test

There are few situations more frustrating to parents than when, the night before a test, their child appears to know the material very well, yet the next day takes the test and scores a 42. What went wrong? During studying, the child's attention is focused with the help of a parent. During a test, however, many more distractions are present in the classroom, and the child is on his own staying focused and recalling information. And often he can't. In addition, the test may take place as long as twenty hours after the child has studied for it, so many distractions have intervened since then.

Spelling tests are frequently an exception because a teacher typically calls out a word, then waits for each child to finish writing it. For this reason, many children with AD/HD perform better on spelling quizzes than they do on other kinds of tests. Moreover, teachers often help children organize the way they study spelling: writing the word several times on Monday, alphabetizing them on Tuesday, using them in sentences on Wednesday, and reviewing them on Thursday before the test on Friday.

Nevertheless, once children start to daydream or become distracted in the midst of a spelling test, they have a hard time regaining their place and often leave out many words or don't complete the last parts of the test.

Responds Inconsistently to Appropriate Incentives

What often stymies parents and teachers about children with AD/HD is the consistency of their inconsistencies. For example, on one occasion, a child might work quickly at cleaning up his room in order to go swimming with his friends. In a similar situation at a different time, however, his parents may find him in his room playing instead of cleaning up. And if asked, "Don't you want to go swimming?" his face might light up as if to say, "Why, of course! Why would you ask such a silly question?" But he also would have to be reminded again about what he needs to do before he can go swimming.

Shows Evidence of Poor Self-Esteem

The way a child feels about himself is reflected in the look on his face, his body language, his motivation to participate in various activities, and the things he says. Indeed, many children with AD/HD look sad and choose not to participate in extracurricular activities. Often this is related to feelings of inadequacy and fear of more failure. More distressing to parents, however, is a child's claims that he is stupid, that nobody likes him, that he hates his parents, or that he'd rather be dead.

An analysis of these statements is complicated. The child who knows that he understands his school work, but continues to make poor grades, thinks he is stupid in spite of what others tell him. This is particularly true when he sees other children getting better grades than he does, even when he is sure that he knows more than they do. Similarly, if the children he wants to play with reject him, his perception is that "nobody" likes him, even when an adult assures him that he does have close friends. From the child's perspective, it's a pretty lousy life. And, if a child shuts down his engine in the early grades due to lack of success, it is very difficult to get it restarted again later.

Is Significantly More Active Than Children of the Same Age

This characteristic identifies children with the hyperactivity component of AD/HD. In young children, hyperactivity may be manifested in constant movement from one place to another, only a few hours of sleep at night, restless sleep, and an inability to sit in one place for more than a few seconds. Hyperactivity tends to decrease as a child approaches adolescence; however, it is typically replaced by more subtle excess movements. As a child gets older, for example, hyperactivity may be characterized more by excessive fidgeting and restlessness. Furthermore, older children often learn to compensate through internal controls, either as a consequence of improved neurological organization or because of increased motivation due to peer pressure or other social or tangible incentives.

Demonstrates Poor Penmanship

Penmanship is a skill that requires a plan for what one wants to write, an understanding of how to put that information on paper, and an ability to transfer that plan to paper. Many children with AD/HD have a great deal of difficulty mastering one or more of these steps. While formulating a plan for what they want to write, for example, they may become distracted and unable to maintain in memory the complete content of what they want to put on paper. Or they may have missed the instructions regarding how it is supposed to go down on paper. Finally, the attention required to the details of putting something down on paper may be so poor that neatness is compromised. Consequently, writing that may start off looking good while attention is high can quickly deteriorate as the child proceeds with the writing task. Letters may become less legible, and the spacing, size, or positioning of the letters and words may be poor. In short, the child may be able to concentrate on the neatness or the content, but not both simultaneously.

Lies or Makes Up Stories

Parents and teachers often report utter frustration with children who have AD/HD because they lie about obvious events. For example, the teacher may see a child take an object from another child's desk and put it in her desk. When confronted, the child denies that she took it and tends to blame someone else or shrug her shoulders. Many children with AD/HD will deny that they have homework, that the teacher told them about a test, or that they took something from school that did not belong to them, for example. While this kind of behavior is characteristic of many young children, appropriate consequences typically cause the behavior to disappear. When the behavior persists in a child with AD/HD, however, it is probably related to the child's impulsiveness. In other words, a youngster with AD/HD will act on an idea that comes to mind without becoming conscious of it. For example, he may see a nice pencil sharpener on another child's desk and say to himself, "I sure wish I had that pencil sharpener." The next thing the child knows, it is in his hand or on his desk, and he never is aware of the process of taking it from the other child's desk!

It is this same lack of conscious monitoring of behavior that causes children with AD/HD to blurt out embarrassing and outrageous statements or to be reported for having their hands all over other children. As a consequence of AD/HD, the child does a poor job monitoring his own behavior and, therefore, may be totally unaware of what he says or does in many instances.

Coexisting Conditions

About two-thirds of children with AD/HD also exhibit one or more other conditions. Many of these are worrisome to parents—and rightfully so. Later in this book, however, we will talk about treatment approaches for AD/HD as well as these coexisting conditions, which should provide more optimism that good outcomes are possible with early diagnosis and prevention.

The most common coexisting psychological conditions with AD/HD are: oppositional defiant disorder (ODD) and conduct disorder (CD), learning disabilities, mood disorders (including depression and bipolar disorder), anxiety disorder, and tics.

The child with ODD argues with adults, blames others, refuses to follow rules, gets angry easily, and frequently annoys others. ODD is found in about 40 percent of children with AD/HD.

Conduct disorders affect about one-quarter of children with AD/HD and are characterized by behaviors usually associated with juvenile delinquency: destroying property, lying and stealing, truancy, and hurting people and animals. Because symptoms often worsen as the child gets older, early identification and treatment is critical. The combination of AD/HD and CD is particularly troublesome, in that children with these untreated coexisting conditions have a very high risk of social and emotional problems in later years. They also are twice as likely to have reading problems than children who have only AD/HD.

As many as half of children with AD/HD also have a learning disability—usually defined as a significant difference between two or more areas of achievement (such as reading, math, or writing) or between an area of achievement and intelligence. The problem is, it's often difficult to determine whether this is a separate problem or one directly related to AD/HD.

Reading disabilities are usually the first to show up, with delays usually occurring in the first and second grades. That's because unlike simple math skills—where children can use their fingers or objects to solve problems—reading requires that a child recognize letter symbols, learn their names and corresponding sounds, and be able to retrieve and combine them on demand. Actually, the foundation for learning to read begins to form well before a child enters kindergarten. The typical child takes notice of shapes, letters, and words and shows an early curiosity about them. The young child with AD/HD, however, may not focus long enough to construct that solid foundation of prereading skills.

Math difficulties, on the other hand, don't usually surface until the introduction of word problems and multiplication and division. That's because these skills require more complex mental calculations and information retrieval than simple addition and subtraction, which a child may have accomplished using his fingers, stroke marks, or objects.

Regardless of subject, only after successful treatment to control the symptoms of AD/HD can one determine if the child has a true learning disability or simply has a learning problem related to the AD/HD.

Mood problems are common, as well, in children with AD/HD. Many of these youngsters appear sad much of the time or show frequent and dramatic swings in mood. Much like learning disabilities, depression may also be a separate problem (it does tend to run in families), or it could be related to the symptoms of AD/HD. For example, a child who is bossy and impulsive is not likely to have many friends. And if being a social outcast is accompanied by disappointing report cards, conflicts at home, and low self-esteem, it's easy for a child to feel sad, rejected, and unsuccessful. As a result, he may say that nobody likes him, or that he would rather be dead.

As a child suffering from AD/HD or depression—or both— gets older, he may be more and more reluctant to participate in group activities. He may also have trouble sleeping or eating and show little enthusiasm for activities he once enjoyed. Some teenagers react to all this by adopting different styles of dress; others might undertake body piercing or even begin cutting themselves.

As many as one in five children with AD/HD also has bipolar disorder. At younger ages, this disorder is characterized by rapid mood changes with no clear reason. The child may act sad and irritable or be combative and aggressive. Unlike adults, in whom cycles of depression and mania can last for days or weeks, children cycle much more rapidly. While mania can be very debilitating as a child gets older, the combination of AD/HD and mania is particularly problematic and can interfere with success in every aspect of life.

About one in ten children with AD/HD also has an anxiety disorder together with AD/HD. While most individuals experience some anxiety and nervousness in particular situations, a child with an anxiety disorder worries excessively, has many unwarranted fears, and feels stressed out or tense much of the time. Some children experience panic attacks, characterized by difficulty breathing, dizziness, a pounding heart, sweating, and fearfulness. Not surprisingly, children with anxiety disorders and AD/HD have more problems in school, at home, and in the community than children who have only AD/HD.

A small number of children with AD/HD also have tics or Tourette's syndrome. Tics are nonpurposeful movements— such as neck stretching, eye scrunching, and lip licking—that occur over and over, and that the child cannot control. Tourette's syndrome is a combination of tics and uncontrolled vocalization, such as sniffing or throat clearing. Stress and fatigue may increase the frequency of the tics.

Some children with AD/HD have obsessions and compulsions, as well. Obsessions are persistent unpleasant thoughts or feelings that interfere with the ability to function normally. Compulsions are ritualistic activities children feel they must engage in before moving on to another activity or continuing with what they were already doing. For example, some youngsters may feel compelled to wash their hands repeatedly after touching a certain object, are driven to follow a certain pattern of behavior before leaving the house, or must place objects in a particular order before feeling at ease. Others must have their food arranged in a certain way on their plate, or they must eat foods in a certain order.

Some children with AD/HD may have a very low tolerance for loud noises or other stimuli. For example, their socks must fit a certain way, or they may be unable to wear shirts with labels that rub against their skin "the wrong way."

Many youngsters with AD/HD are persistent bedwetters, a condition called enuresis. While only about 10 percent of children in the normal population continue to wet the bed at night beyond the age of six, this problem tends to be over-represented in the population of children with AD/HD. Moreover, the most common behavior approaches used to curb bedwetting—reducing fluid intake after dinner, having the child empty his bladder before he goes to bed and again before his parents turn in—yield little consistent success in children with AD/HD. Even use of the popular bell and pad method is only moderately successful for these youngsters and may only add to the stresses the child and his family are experiencing. With this method, a special pad is placed under the sheet. When it is wet by urine, a bell connected to the pad rings. This awakens the child, who can then get up and complete urinating in the toilet.

As mentioned earlier, many children with AD/HD also show signs of depression that may be related to feelings of despair brought on by inability to meet their own—or others'—expectations. It is painful for parents to see their children so unhappy. It is even more painful for the child to live a life characterized by feelings of helplessness and hopelessness. That's why careful diagnosis of AD/HD is necessary. It can help determine if a child's depression has resulted from a specific event—such as a parental divorce, death of a family member, or a serious fight with a best friend—or from more global factors such as continual underachievement as a result of symptoms of AD/HD.

Lisa's story is an excellent example. Lisa is a fourth-grader who consistently makes A's and B's on her report card and who rarely has her name put on the board for misbehaving. Lisa is also a popular child with lots of friends. For the past week or so, however, Lisa has made low D's on the majority of her tests and has failed to turn in her homework most mornings. Her name has been put on the board at least twice every day for talking back to the teacher, and on the playground she has been repeatedly reprimanded for pushing and yelling at her friends.

Lisa's teacher tried talking to her, but Lisa insisted that nothing was wrong. When the teacher threatened to call Lisa's parents, the child became defiant. "Fine," she said. "I don't care. They're not home anyway!"

When her teacher called Lisa's parents to schedule a conference, a baby-sitter reported that they were indeed out of town. Lisa's grandmother—with whom the child had been very close—had just died, and Lisa's parents had gone out of town for two weeks to attend the funeral and to help take care of Lisa's grandfather.

Once the teacher approached Lisa about her grandmother's death, Lisa burst into tears and apologized for misbehaving and not doing her work. The school counselor spent several hours with Lisa over the next few weeks and Lisa soon returned to her old self.

Summary

Children with AD/HD are a diverse group. They are affected by biological, hereditary, and environmental factors that researchers are still trying to unravel. Many children have problems beyond AD/HD, which may have further dramatic impact on their successful performance in school, at home, and in the community—both in the near and long term.

It's up to parents to be alert to the first signs and symptoms of AD/HD—and experts agree these may show up as early as infancy and toddlerhood in the form of frequent temper tantrums, severe separation anxiety, constant refusals to go to sleep, and other unruly behavior. Yet, sadly, studies show that most youngsters go a full decade before they are properly diagnosed with this treatable disorder.

Successful treatment of AD/HD requires that a team of professionals work together, which can be overwhelming for parents. But the good news is that early diagnosis, intervention, and treatment have been shown to help these youngsters overcome their problems and achieve success in all areas of their life.

CHAPTER 2

DOES MY CHILD HAVE AD/HD?

Alicia, now ten, was held back a year when she was in kindergarten. Her teacher felt that Alicia was "immature" and would do best if she had another year in kindergarten to mature. It was during that first year in kindergarten that Alicia, her mother, and her younger brother and sister moved out of their home and into a shelter for protection from Alicia's abusive father. Alicia's mother got a job at a grocery store, where her work hours required that her younger children be in a daycare center most of the day. Alicia went to the daycare center before school and often after school as well.

During Alicia's second year in kindergarten, her performance improved very little. Her teacher indicated that Alicia was refusing to do work, spent much of her time wandering around the room, and frequently bickered with other children. "I am sure she has all of the right skills," the teacher reported to Alicia's mother. "It is just so hard to get them out of her."

Her mother described Alicia as very defiant and

obstinate around the house—"Always trying to tell
me what to do," she said. The family moved into an
apartment soon after Alicia's second year of kinder-
garten began. Alicia's mother hoped that things would
settle down once her family's life became more stable.
But Alicia's problems in school and at home persisted.

Alicia is now in the third grade at the age of ten, and
her problems still have not disappeared. Her mother
recently got a better job that allows her to spend more
time with the children. Still, there have been no im-
provements in Alicia's school performance, and her
behavior at home has become even more explosive
and defiant.

Maybe your child hasn't been professionally diagnosed as having AD/HD, but you sense that something is wrong. Or maybe she's been tested in school and has been described as having characteristics consistent with AD/HD, but no treatment was recommended. Should you seek professional advice? There are questions you should ask yourself to determine if your child meets the criteria for pursuing additional help:

- Does my child daydream often and seem to be distracted easily when she is involved in an activity at home?
- Does my child have trouble sitting quietly long enough to complete her homework unless I sit with her?
- Does my child begin projects and activities but lose interest in them before they are completed?
- Does my child have difficulty following my directions?
- Does my child have difficulty sitting still at meals, for homework, in restaurants, and in church or synagogue?
- Does my child have trouble making and keeping friends who are the same age as he is?

- Is my child argumentative and does she interrupt me constantly when I am on the phone or talking to friends?
- Does my child seem to know school material when we study together but perform poorly on tests of the same material?
- Does my child often forget to write down her homework assignments or forget to bring home the necessary books to complete homework or studying?
- Does my child have trouble making and keeping friends?

If you answered yes to many of these questions and your child exhibits this behavior frequently, you owe it to your child and yourself to discuss your concerns with your child's physician. In turn, the physician may request that you involve either a private psychologist (preferably one who specializes in AD/HD) or the school psychologist and support staff. Otherwise, if she does have AD/HD and her disorder is left unrecognized and untreated, the problems she is experiencing now may only become worse.

The Great Impostors: When It's Not AD/HD

Up until fifth grade, Karen breezed through school. Her grades were always well above average and her teacher always remarked to her parents what a joy Karen was to teach. About a month into fifth grade, however, everything changed. Karen's grades began slipping and she was often singled out in the classroom for not paying attention. She rarely turned her homework in on time and began ignoring her friends on the playground, preferring instead to play by herself. When her teacher asked Karen what was wrong, she hung her head and said, "Nothing."

Concerned, her teacher set up a conference with Karen's parents and discovered that the two had recently separated. Her parents acknowledged that they knew Karen was upset about the situation, but admitted that they'd been so busy arguing that they weren't aware of how deeply their marital problems had affected their daughter.

A number of factors can cause symptoms that mimic AD/HD, and these should be addressed or ruled out as causes before treating a child for the disorder.

Family Problems

Marital discord. Divorce. A family death. Substance abuse. Child abuse. Sexual molestation. These are just a few situations that can cause AD/HD-like behavior to surface in children. In many cases, however, youngsters bounce back once the stressful situation is alleviated, or they learn to cope with the stress, and needed counseling is provided. In Karen's case, for example, once her parents realized the toll their behavior was taking on their daughter, they sought family counseling to learn how best to handle their impending divorce. After several therapy sessions, Karen's behavior returned to normal. When a child's problem behavior is chronic, however, AD/HD is often the culprit.

Learning Disabilities

Youngsters who have difficulty processing information due to a learning disability may appear less interested in what people are saying or in school-related work. Those with mental handicaps or learning disabilities may also give up easily on tasks or become resigned to being "behavior problems," since structured activities with normal expectations tend to be less satisfying. For this reason, it is important to have your child's learning and perceptual abilities evaluated before accepting a diagnosis of AD/HD.

In fact, most schools will include academic screening as part of the evaluation process. This type of screening provides important information about a child's intelligence and achievement (for example, reading and math skills) and can be extremely beneficial in that it may suggest the possibility of an intellectual deficit or a learning disability. Academic screening can also rule out the need for a full battery of psychological tests, which can be time-consuming and costly when performed by a private psychologist.

Chuck's story is a good example. When Chuck, an average student, began failing in third grade, his parents scheduled a conference with his teacher. "We went over all of his papers and discovered that he was copying a lot of questions and math problems from the chalkboard incorrectly. Consequently, he was getting a lot of the wrong answers," his mother explains. "Most of the time, it seemed like he was copying numbers and some words and letters backward."

Chuck's parents suspected that their son was just being lazy and careless, but asked the school to test him anyway. "As it turns out, Chuck had a learning disability," his mother says. "Now he's enrolled in special classes and his grades are improving."

Sensory Problems

When a child has trouble seeing the chalkboard or when blurred vision prevents her from being able to read assignments or classwork, she may fidget in her seat, turn in careless work, or be mislabeled as inattentive or lazy. Other vision problems can also masquerade as AD/HD. When researchers at the University of California–San Diego's Shiley Eye Center recently reviewed records of seventeen hundred children diagnosed with AD/HD, they discovered that of those who had taken eye exams, 16 percent had convergence insufficiency, an eye disorder that makes focusing on nearby objects difficult. Naturally, youngsters with this disorder can find reading a real struggle. And since doctors often test for AD/HD by examining reading comprehension, this creates obvious potential for misdiagnosis.

Hearing impairments can also cause problems, such as difficulty with communication or inability to pay attention. A child who can't hear well, for example, may appear uninterested or as if he's not listening. He may also be labeled forgetful or inattentive when he simply didn't hear instructions correctly.

Thyroid Dysfunction

Many symptoms of thyroid dysfunction are identical to those of AD/HD and include depression, sadness, and an inability to concentrate. (See Chapter Three for more details on this connection.)

Lead Toxicity

When low but toxic levels of lead in children go undetected, their language skills suffer. So do their cognitive abilities and short-term memory—and they often have trouble staying focused on tasks. Lead toxicity is most often found in children exposed to lead-based paint and water transported through old lead pipes.

Sleep Disorders

Lack of proper sleep can frequently result in AD/HD-like symptoms: inability to sustain attention, decreased ability to follow directions, fuzzy thinking, and a tendency to drift off during conversations. Recent evidence suggests that even sleep-disordered breathing, such as heavy snoring, can be equally problematic—particularly in boys under eight years of age. Daytime problems often improve, however, once these sleep problems are treated.

Emily's story is a good example. When her teacher called Emily's parents to report that the fourth-grader wasn't paying attention in class, Emily's mom was surprised. "No teacher had ever said that about our daughter," says Emily's mom, Beth. "In fact, lots of her teachers in past years had told us just the opposite—that Emily was always raising her hand to ask and answer questions in class. So, right away, I knew something was wrong and made Emily an appointment with our pediatrician."

Following a sleep study, Emily was diagnosed with sleep apnea, a condition in which people stop breathing every couple of minutes while sleeping—sometimes for more than thirty seconds before twitching and gasping. "We now realize that, because Emily wasn't sleeping well at night, she was exhausted at school and showing signs of hyperactivity in an effort to stay awake!" says Beth. "Within two weeks after getting treated, Emily was sleeping soundly again, and all her teachers agreed her improvement was remarkable."

Seizures

They may last just a few seconds and be so mild a child doesn't even notice them. Yet, since certain types of seizures (petit mal or absence seizures) cause brief staring episodes, they can be misunderstood as inattention, poor listening skills, or an inability to concentrate.

Nutritional Deficiencies

Iron levels that are too low can cause irritability, lack of concentration, shortened attention span, and impaired cognitive skills—all symptoms found in children with AD/HD. The same can be said for reactive hypoglycemia—or low blood sugar—which causes the body to respond with a rapid rush of insulin that can lead to hyperactivity and irritability.

Parenting/Caregiving Styles

The approach that parents and other caregivers use to raise and discipline a child—and the consistency among caregivers—can have a major impact on a youngster's behavior. For children with AD/HD, a good match with a caregiving style is particularly important.

For example, if a caregiver has an *authoritarian* style—or rules with an iron hand—the child will have few opportunities to make her own decisions. Moreover, this kind of caregiver usually takes a "spare the rod and spoil the child" approach when it comes to disciplining youngsters, which translates into punishing children (often severely) when they break any of the many rules to which they are expected to adhere.

Children with *permissive* caregivers, on the other hand, tend to have free rein to set their own rules. This kind of caregiver places few limits on the child, believing that she will learn best by pursuing her own interests and satisfying her own curiosity. What often happens instead is that permissive caregivers eventually become resigned to the fact that they have a difficult child on their hands and that few disciplinary measures seem to work. Consequently, they often give up by taking a *laissez-faire* approach with the child, and everyone else who must deal with the child is forced to suffer the consequences.

Finally, the *authoritative* caregiver sets clear limits but is willing to negotiate those limits in certain instances. For example, if a child's bedtime is eight-thirty, but a special show is on TV that doesn't end until nine, an authoritative parent might allow the child to stay up later. However, the parent would also make it clear to the child that her regular bedtime would return the next evening. Authoritative caregivers also make it a point to give their children opportunities to make decisions and to help them understand the consequences for making right and wrong decisions.

How do caregiving styles affect children's behavior? Research indicates that children of authoritarian and permissive caregivers tend to do more poorly in school and in life. At one extreme, children are not given the opportunity to make their own decisions; thus they may make decisions poorly when put in the position of having to structure themselves. At the other extreme is the child who has grown up in a permissive environment in which she has not had to adapt to social rules. Consequently, in a structured daycare or school environment where there are specific expectations for her performance, she has difficulty conforming to rules.

Consistency in caregiving styles is also important. When rules change constantly or when children are forced to deal with caregivers who have different expectations for them, they become confused and often manipulative.

Matt's story is a good example. Matt is ten years old and has a history of talking back to his parents and being defiant in school with teachers and administrators. In addition, he has had many explosive outbursts both at school and at home. Matt's parents have tried many behavior management strategies over the years, ranging from verbal reprimand to yelling and spanking. None of these has worked; in fact, Matt's episodes of poor behavior have increased over time.

After talking to a psychologist, Matt's parents implemented a program at home that was very rigid and structured. Under the plan, Matt lost part of his allowance and television time for each outburst and episode of talking back. The management program was begun during the summer, when there was consistent contact between Matt and his parents.

Over the course of just a few weeks, both Matt and his parents acknowledged great improvement in his ability to demonstrate self-control. Initially, he became apologetic after his outbursts or episodes of talking back. Then he started catching himself in the middle of the behavior and was able to interrupt and subdue it. Finally, he showed an overall decrease in the number of such episodes.

When Matt's parents returned to talk to the psychologist, they indicated great concern about how both sets of grandparents were unsupportive of their efforts. The grandparents let Matt get away with talking back and excused the behavior as Matt's being "just a boy." Often they would contradict Matt's parents in front of him. His parents reported that it often took

Matt several days to return to an improved level of behavior after visiting with his grandparents.

In addition to having to deal with the effects that the varying caregiving styles had on their son, Matt's parents were faced with the dilemma of either putting up with the unpleasant consequences of his behavior following a visit with his grandparents or giving the grandparents an ultimatum to change their approach or not see Matt.

Temperament

Temperament refers to a child's innate personality, which can range from easygoing, to slow to warm up, to difficult. While temperament is determined by genetics and neurochemical makeup, some components of temperament—and, later, personality—can be modified by a child's environment. Many children who show difficult behavior patterns as infants—including colic, irregular sleep and feeding patterns, and persistent fussiness—may be easy to care for and agreeable once they grow up. On the other hand, children who are easy to care for as infants may become more difficult to handle as time passes. While a difficult temperament may affect aspects of the child's behavior and learning, it does not always predict AD/HD. It is important to differentiate between specific characteristics of AD/HD and those of a difficult temperament before establishing a treatment plan.

Fatigue, Illness, and Hunger

Behavior changes are common when any of us feels tired, hungry, or ill, and this is particularly true for children. Those with greater need for sleep or those who tend to have irregular eating habits may be tired or hungry more often during the day. Often, changes in their behavior are simply a consequence of these factors. For example, the first-grader who becomes wild and uncontrollable periodically may be having a difficult time coping without the nap she was used to taking at home or in kindergarten last year. The cumulative effect of sleep deprivation can cause problems as well.

Youngsters who are prone to middle-ear infections, constipation, or similar chronic problems may also show alterations in behavior as a result of their discomfort. Therefore, it is important to rule out life pattern factors and chronic illnesses as possible causes of behavior before considering a diagnosis of AD/HD.

Diet

While changes in behavior have been reported for many children in response to certain diet products and foods (such as sweets), researchers have found little evidence to support this claim. And there is scant evidence that allergies to other environmental substances may alter a child's behavior. Unfortunately, many unfounded claims and theories have received a great deal of national publicity on television talk shows and in tabloids. As a result, viewers are often led to believe that there is sound scientific evidence to support these claims. In fact, there is none.

Nevertheless the wealth of anecdotal reports of children whose behavior has improved dramatically with the elimination of certain foods makes diet an important consideration for children with behavior and learning problems. Thus parents should begin by observing the child's short-term behavior following eating or drinking certain substances. In addition, they might try decreasing, one at a time, the common allergenic products in the child's diet that the child consumes in large quantities—for example, chocolate, tomato products, eggs, and milk.

If a child has a history of allergies or is congested at certain times during the year, your physician may recommend allergy testing. However, in general, although allergic responses to foods or environmental substances may make an attention problem worse, they are rarely the cause of the problem.

Teacher-Child Mismatch

Unfortunately, there are times when a teacher's style clashes with a child's temperament and learning style. And sometimes, neither adjustment by the teacher nor adaptation by the child can solve the problem. Of course, not every teacher your child has will be outstanding. Nevertheless, parents hope that their children will be resilient enough to accommodate a teacher's personality and teaching style. But not all children have this resilience. In fact, some teachers may be so difficult for a child to accommodate to that the stress of this daily confrontation may elicit somatic complaints (for example, headaches and stomachaches) from the child, as well as symptoms that mimic AD/HD.

What can parents do in such situations? Most schools have an informal policy of not changing a child's class once school starts. But by taking an assertive approach to the problem, you may be able to convince school administrators to bend the rules. Keep in mind, though, that school administrators must deal with many children's needs; a request for a change of teachers should be made only for sound educational reasons— and only after other approaches have failed.

To begin your campaign, gather documentation to prove that your child has a history of good performance in school and is capable of doing the work, but is so distressed by the teacher's approach that her work productivity has suffered. Make an appointment to present your argument and documentation to the school administrator. If she refuses to consider your request, let her know that you intend to call or show up in person with any and all new information about your child's problems in school until the move is made! Be pleasant and cordial, but also firm and persistent. Your child's present and future success may be at stake, and that is something worth fighting for.

As a parent of a child with AD/HD, it is critical that you play the role of advocate. You can best do this by educating yourself and others about this common disorder, by doing whatever you can to minimize the stress your child experiences, and by helping others who interact with your child regularly to do the same.

To Test or Not to Test

When children have behavior or learning problems, parents are often advised by a number of sources to have their youngsters tested for academic and psychological strengths and weaknesses. Parents have the option of having the school system test the child (at no cost to them) or having tests administered privately (which can cost in excess of a thousand dollars). Schools are usually reluctant to test children unless there is significant evidence of learning problems. That's because procedures for testing through the school system are time-consuming and involve wading through many complex bureaucratic steps, both before testing and for follow-up information. Nevertheless, if your child is having problems and you want to find out what's wrong, don't let these drawbacks dissuade you.

In fact, federal education laws require school systems to test any child who is three years of age or older who might be eligible for special education services.

Psychological and academic testing can be particularly useful for several types of children. First, it may benefit those who show particular strengths and particular weaknesses in their academic work. In other words, when a child performs above average in some area of academics but does very poorly in others, this may indicate a learning disability that may either accompany AD/HD or be a consequence of poor attention during the early years.

Second, testing can be useful for children who show generalized delays in all academic areas. Again, this developmental delay may accompany AD/HD or be a consequence of it. Nevertheless, if the delays are significant enough, the child may be eligible for additional remedial education through the schools.

Finally, testing may be useful in pinpointing a significant social or emotional problem demonstrated in the educational setting. In this case, projective testing and various types of rating scales are used to identify the type of, and sometimes the reason for, the social and emotional problems.

Formal psychological testing of children is a lengthy process that may involve several hours of contact between the psychologist and the child, often over the course of several days. Testing generally involves measures of intelligence (common tests in this area include the Wechsler Intelligence Scale for Children, the Stanford-Binet Intelligence Test, and the Kaufman Assessment Battery for Children) and measures of academic achievement (the Peabody Individual Achievement Test, the Kaufman Test of Education Achievement, the Woodcock-Johnson Tests of Achievement, and the Wechsler Individual Achievement Test are most common), and may involve measures of emotional status, specific language skills, and perceptual-motor skills.

School Services Available and Your Rights as a Parent

In most cases, a recommendation to have a child tested through a school program is made by the Student Support Team (see page 115)—and only after trying many other approaches to help a child in the educational setting. As a parent, you must give written consent for the testing. You also have a right to review the results of all testing that is done.

If you agree to have your child tested, don't do anything or treat him any differently to prepare him for the procedure.

In other words, don't put him to bed earlier than usual. Also avoid prompting him or giving him medication he would not normally take. You want the psychologist to see your child in his typical state—demonstrating skills and exhibiting behavior that are representative of how he normally performs and behaves in the classroom—except, of course, that testing is generally done on a one-to-one basis.

Following the testing, you will be invited in for a conference to discuss various options based on your child's test results. If these indicate that your child qualifies for special education services, you will have an opportunity to learn about and consider the type and extent of services he needs. Keep in mind that special education services for eligible children are based on what a child *needs* rather than what services are currently being provided by the school. Therefore, if there is evidence of a severe problem, more intensive intervention should be prescribed.

Schools are required by federal law to follow the principle of Least Restrictive Environment, which supports the idea that children with special needs should be served in a setting that is as close to normal as possible while simultaneously meeting their educational needs. If the school recommends special education services for your child—or if you feel that special services are needed but the school does not make those recommendations—you have many rights for due process to question or appeal the school's decision. To keep this process as productive and cordial as possible, however, it is often wise to discuss your options with a professional or another knowledgeable parent who will serve as your and your child's advocate.

There will be decisions to make every step of the way. First, you'll need to decide whether to have your child tested. Second, if he is tested, you must decide if you feel the test results accurately reflect your child's ability—and if not, decide what recourse you have. Then you need to decide whether to accept special education placement if your child is eligible. If he is not eligible for special services, you must decide whether to accept the decision or to appeal it. If he is eligible, you must decide, together with school personnel, on the best placement for your child. There are a range of options here: modifications in the regular classroom, part-time placement in a resource class, full-time placement in a special education class, placement in a special facility for children with the type of problem your child is experiencing, and so on. Finally, you'll need to decide on specific goals and objectives that the program should strive to achieve with your child.

Decisions, decisions. If you find yourself feeling confused, overwhelmed, and fearful of making the wrong choices, find a knowledgeable friend, a professional, or a member of your local AD/HD support group to assist you with these important decisions. And bear in mind that you can rescind your consent at any time if you realize later that a particular decision might not be in your child's best interest.

Some parents consider home-schooling their youngsters. Granted, home-schooling may provide more opportunities for the child to feel successful, offer a more distraction-free environment, and provide the one-to-one teaching by which she is likely to learn best, but it may also be counterproductive. Unless there are also opportunities built into the child's schedule for social and recreational activities with peers, her learning may suffer in several dimensions. Moreover, if interactions between a parent and a child have tended to be unpleasant, home-schooling can easily increase both the parent's and the child's levels of frustration.

Other parents consider transferring their child to private school. Youngsters with AD/HD often improve in private-school settings because of smaller class sizes and greater opportunities for one-on-one interactions with their teachers.

But this option is almost always an expensive one that many parents simply cannot afford. And often the academic challenges and work demands are greater.

In Chapter Seven, we specifically address strategies and issues related to working with the schools in a productive way. Given that youngsters spend about one-fifth of their childhood in school, this home away from home must be conducive to learning and good behavior.

3

WHAT WE KNOW
ABOUT THE CAUSES OF AD/HD

David, a sixth-grader, is an adopted child who has always struggled academically. Since kindergarten his teachers have described him as easily distracted and as having a short attention span. But, they add, he is usually a very sociable and pleasant child.

This year, David had detention numerous times, primarily for coming to class unprepared and for wandering the halls without a pass. And recently he was suspended for two days after getting into a fistfight with another child.

At home, David's parents say he rarely appears motivated to do school work and that he never lets them know when he has homework or exams. Because of this lack of communication, his parents claim they are unable to monitor their son's progress or help him prepare for tests.

David spends most of his time at home listening to music and reading. Despite his academic and

*behavioral problems, he says he likes school. None-
theless, David appears to be on a course that can only
lead to increasing problems both at school and at
home.*

Whose Fault Is It?

Whenever children have problems, there's a natural tendency
to look for something or someone to blame for their misfor-
tune. In David's case, one might point the finger at his parents, arguing that they appear too permissive. After all, what
"good" parents rely on a child to tell them when he has a test
or when an important assignment is due? If a child were failing, wouldn't it make more sense for the parents to check with
the child's teacher about his assignments? Furthermore, when
a youngster is sent to detention as often as David has been and
has been suspended for fighting as well, doesn't this suggest a
lack of discipline on the home front?

On the other hand, David is adopted. And since AD/HD is
known to have genetic roots, perhaps he has inherited the disorder from one of his biological parents.

Then again, maybe David's teachers are partly to blame.
After all, he appears to have been labeled impulsive and easily
distracted since kindergarten. And since children can usually
sense how others—particularly adults—perceive them, they
often develop self-concepts to meet the expectations others
have of them. If this is true in David's case, he is likely caught
in a vicious cycle. Because his teachers perceive him as a
low achiever and a behavior problem, he has little self-esteem.
This, in turn, can easily lead to poor social-adjustment skills,
developmental delays, and academic failure. Indeed, there is a
degree of self-fulfilling prophecy related to AD/HD for a child
who is unable to live up to anyone's expectations in an environment that does not conform to the child's needs. In other
words, unless the cycle is interrupted, failure begets failure.

AD/HD can leave *everyone* involved feeling frustrated. The child performs poorly even when he is motivated and putting forth his best effort. Parents feel incompetent because the child is not responding to their attempts at consistent behavior management and childrearing approaches. Teachers feel frustrated and inadequate because all the approaches they learned in school and at workshops have proven unsuccessful at getting one particular child to perform to his potential.

All of this paints a bleak picture—one in which everyone involved feels despondent, unsatisfied, and even responsible for the dilemma. But the truth is, no one individual is to blame for the child's problems, although the behavior patterns of parents, teachers, and the child himself can certainly aggravate the situation. In fact, research indicates that the major source of dramatic social and academic problems in a child with AD/HD is biological in nature.

Nature or Nurture?

Compelling evidence suggests that in some cases, at least, genetic factors may contribute to AD/HD. In fact, some family studies have found that parents, children, or brothers or sisters of someone with the disorder have a fivefold greater risk of AD/HD than someone in the general population. Many readers may have already realized that they—or a spouse—exhibited many of the characteristics of AD/HD in their youth and may still exhibit them today. (For this reason, we have devoted a chapter later in this book to AD/HD in adulthood.) All of this reinforces the idea that the cause of AD/HD is biological. But not every case of AD/HD is attributable to heredity.

What else might cause AD/HD? In some cases, clues can be found in a child's environment. These include premature birth, maternal alcohol and tobacco use, lead exposure in early childhood, psychosocial adversity, and brain injuries. These factors account for about 20 to 30 percent of AD/HD in boys and a slightly smaller percentage in girls. However, research has found no links between AD/HD and poor parenting, vitamin deficiencies, allergies, excessive sugar intake, or exposure to radiation.

The Brain Connection

Many studies have clearly pointed to differences in the structure and chemical functioning of parts of the brain in children with AD/HD. For example, in one decade-long study conducted by the National Institutes of Health in Bethesda, researchers took magnetic resonance imaging (MRI) brain images of both children diagnosed with AD/HD and youngsters who did not have the disorder. Their findings have produced some fascinating revelations.

By first grade, the human brain is 90 to 95 percent the size of the adult brain. However, refinement of the structures of the brain continues through adolescence. The size of the brain can vary greatly from one person to the next at any given age. Nevertheless, children with AD/HD have slightly smaller brain volume overall (about 5 percent). Several areas of the brain appear to be consistently smaller in youngsters with AD/HD— the basal ganglia (a part that lies deep within the brain and has many responsibilities we will discuss later), the corpus callosum (the part of the brain that connects the right and left lobes of the cerebrum), and a part of the cerebellum called the vermis. In addition, there are consistent differences in the sizes of right and left parts of the brain of typical individuals. But these relationships do not hold up for children with AD/HD for important brain parts, such as the prefrontal cortex.

The prefrontal cortex lies just behind the forehead and is referred to as the "executive" part of the brain. It is wired to virtually every system in the brain and plays a critical role in every aspect of our ability to learn, stay focused on a task, pull things we need out of memory, and respond to our environment.

Perhaps Yale University researcher Thomas E. Brown, Ph.D., explained it best when he compared the executive part of the brain to the conductor of an orchestra. "Picture a symphony where all the musicians are good," Brown says. "But if the conductor cannot get them to play their respective parts at the same time, you are not going to get very good music. The problem with AD/HD is not with the individual musicians; the problem is essentially with the conductor."

Much of the original research that first identified how the brain works differently in children with AD/HD, as compared to typical children, used a procedure called Positron Emission Tomography (PET) to provide a dynamic picture of brain activity. This procedure allows researchers to look at how quickly oxygen is metabolized in various parts of the brain, which indicates the level of activity in these parts. For example, when a person is reading, the visual cortex—the part of the brain responsible for interpreting visual material—appears most active, while other areas of the brain appear less active. Similarly, when a person is listening to music with his eyes closed, the auditory cortex of the brain appears very active, while other areas appear less active. These images are pictured on a computer screen with color enhancement to differentiate activity levels by different colors and shades.

The PET scan procedure has been used in research to identify brain differences in individuals with many types of suspected brain disorders. To date, it has revealed differences between normal individuals and those with depression, schizophrenia, Alzheimer's disease, obsessive-compulsive disorder, and others.

This approach also has been used with individuals with AD/HD to identify the specific parts of the brain that appear to be performing differently from the typical individual. And it is those parts of the prefrontal cortex and associated brain areas that show less activity than would be expected based on the brain activity of typical children.

How does this play out in a real-world situation? In a classroom setting, for example, when this area of the frontal lobe is functioning normally, a child can easily pay attention to the teacher, concentrate on the work in front of him, or focus on the announcement he hears over the loudspeaker. He can copy down his homework assignment accurately and stay in his seat while his classmate gets up to get a drink from the water fountain. However, when this part of the brain is not functioning normally, all incoming information tends to compete on an equal basis. In other words, the brain is unable to prioritize the most important information coming in and to filter out "noise"—a nearby child shuffling papers at his seat, a truck rumbling by outside the window, the smells of lunch being prepared down the hall, or a group of classmates reading aloud in the corner of the room. In the child with AD/HD, all of these stimuli receive the same attention from the brain as the worksheet sitting on the child's desk that he is supposed to be working on.

Furthermore, this "executive" part of the brain is *supposed* to inhibit activity in other parts of the brain that aren't needed to accomplish a specific task at hand. For example, when a child needs to sit still to complete an assignment, the "executive" part of the brain should limit activity in the motor (movement) area of the brain. The problem is, when the prefrontal cortex doesn't do its job, no brakes are available to control interference with learning. So, the child may be fidgety, distractible, impulsive, and talkative.

The Chemical Connection

Long before all of this extensive research on the structural differences of the brain, scientists began paying careful attention to the role of certain brain chemicals, called neurotransmitters, in AD/HD. That research continues, and this much we know: These chemicals are important for two reasons. First, some neurotransmitters help nerve impulses move efficiently across the synaptic gaps between each of the billions of nerve cells in the brain. Second, other neurotransmitters *block* the passage of certain nerve impulses across the synapses to prevent unwanted movements—for example, when remaining absolutely still is necessary.

Several of these neurotransmitters have become the focus of intense scrutiny since they communicate information in parts of the brain that are responsible for alertness, attention, and freedom from distractions. Collectively, these particular neurotransmitters are called catecholamines and include dopamine and norepinephrine. There is a strong belief that AD/HD symptoms are a result of a deficiency of dopamine and, indirectly, norepinephrine—particularly in the prefrontal cortex area. Naturally, low levels of these chemicals would be expected to cause decreased activity in that part of the brain, as well as corresponding symptoms we see in children with AD/HD—including short attention span, distractibility, hyperactivity, poor impulse control, difficulty retrieving learned material, poor organization, and emotional inconsistencies. In fact, the two genes that have been implicated in AD/HD are those that play a role in governing the effectiveness of how dopamine works in the brain.

So what happens to these neurotransmitters that makes things go haywire in the brain and leads to utter chaos in some children's performance and behavior? Recent research conducted at New York's Brookhaven National Laboratory found that the brains of youngsters with AD/HD have too little dopamine. "Dopamine is not only involved with movement and attention, but with reward and motivation," reports study author Nora Volkow, M.D. "It modulates brain signals that say, 'This is important. Pay attention!'"

For this message to be received, however, nerve impulses

must be able to move efficiently from nerve cell to nerve cell, and for them to do that, dopamine must first fill in the spaces between nerve cells. Then, once dopamine is released into the synapse, it must bind with target receptors on the next nerve cell. Otherwise, it is reabsorbed into the nerve cell and important messages never get through.

According to Dr. Volkow's research, the brains of children with AD/HD have too many molecules that suck up dopamine before it can do its job. In other words, in these youngsters, there appears to be a defect in this binding process, and dopamine does not remain in the synapse long enough. Instead, it is reabsorbed into the nerve cell.

Another neurotransmitter, serotonin, is suspected of playing a role in the emotional aspects of AD/HD. As with the catecholamines, an absence of available serotonin in the synapses appears to be responsible for AD/HD symptoms.

The result? A disorganized pattern of attention and arousal, often inefficient processing of information in various parts of the brain responsible for handling visual and auditory information, problems retrieving information from memory, and, in some cases, uncontrolled and disorganized movement patterns.

The implications of this problem with the brain can be profound. Aside from making decisions about what incoming information is important and should be attended to—as opposed to information that is best ignored—the prefrontal cortex also controls what parts of the brain should be activated to efficiently process important incoming information. For example, if a child is taking a test, the visual cortex of his brain and areas of memory storage would most likely be activated. At the same time, the prefrontal cortex would inhibit activity in the auditory cortex so that he would not be distracted by noises around him during the test. In individuals with AD/HD, however, this efficient process does not occur. Therefore, parts of the brain that should be inhibited—such as the motor area—may not be. The result: a child who fidgets and changes position often during an activity when he should be sitting still.

In the broader picture, the inability of the coordinating center of the child's brain to control thinking and movement causes him to be inconsistent, impulsive, and out of control. And it is these factors that create the severe level of frustration that everyone in the child's environment—including the child himself—experiences.

Here's a good analogy to help you empathize with your AD/HD child. Remember what it's like to carry on a conversation with someone at a loud party or in a noisy restaurant? It can be difficult to hear the person you're talking to because, while you're trying to listen to her, you are being bombarded with other sights and sounds that are competing on an equal basis. So you strain and struggle to focus on what is being said but are often unsuccessful—right?

What's happening here is that the brain is trying to sort out the important sounds from all the other competing sounds but is having a difficult time doing so. Essentially, all the stimuli in your environment are competing for your attention on the same level, and your brain is failing in its task to help you sort out the important information.

The lives of children with AD/HD appear to follow this pattern. The assignment on the board that must be copied down is competing for attention with a conglomeration of other sights and sounds, as well as other thoughts that are racing through the child's head. As a result, the child has difficulty following instructions, completing assignments, controlling unnecessary movements, retrieving information for tests and discussions, and processing information appropriately.

We do not know why children with AD/HD can concentrate efficiently at certain times but not at others. We do know, though, that the inconsistencies and general patterns of difficulty are frustrating for these children as well as for everyone around them. Indeed, these dysfunctions interfere not only with the child's ability to read, write, and solve mathematical problems, but also with his ability to get along with his peers and family members.

The Thyroid Connection

Several years ago, researchers at the National Institute for Diabetes and Digestive and Kidney Diseases in Bethesda found that children suffering from a rare genetic disease—resistance to thyroid hormone—also showed a very high rate of AD/HD. When a specific gene works correctly, a particular protein in the body responds to thyroid hormone and helps control metabolism and heart rate as well as brain development in the fetus. However, when this gene is defective, the protein performs abnormally. This may result in short stature, enlargement of the thyroid gland, cardiac problems, and AD/HD. In fact, about 70 percent of children and half of adults with thyroid hormone resistance show symptoms of AD/HD.

Someday soon, this discovery will likely play a role in early identification of individuals with thyroid hormone resistance, who then stand a good chance of developing AD/HD. Unfortunately, however, it is unlikely that this discovery will lead to any cure for AD/HD in the near future—either for the very small percentage of the population with thyroid hormone resistance or for those individuals who show symptoms of AD/HD.

Nevertheless, this finding provides further reinforcement that AD/HD is biologically based. Many physicians are now checking thyroid function as part of their AD/HD diagnostic process. Treatment of this condition with artificial thyroid hormone can alleviate many of the accompanying symptoms of AD/HD. As time passes, more and more will be learned about causes of AD/HD, with the hope that, at some time in the near future, scientists will have the knowledge and technology to eradicate this disorder.

CHAPTER

4

THE IMPACT OF AD/HD

All of his life, Jason has loathed school. "We held him back in the fifth grade, but he continued to struggle after that," says Jason's mom, Lois. "And over the years, his teachers have always complained about his disruptive behavior." At seventeen, Jason decided to drop out of high school.

That was a year ago. Since then, Jason has bounced from one low-paying job to another—usually getting fired because of his lackluster attitude. His number one wish at the moment is to move out of his parents' home, but he can't afford to pay for his own apartment right now.

In his early teen years, Jason got in trouble with the law twice. "At fourteen, he was charged with underage drinking," Lois reports. "At sixteen, he got caught with marijuana and served thirty days at a juvenile detention center."

Not surprisingly, Jason's relationship with his parents is tense. Nor does he have any close friends. "He has had a couple of girlfriends, but these relationships rarely last longer than a month," adds Lois, who now suspects that her son has AD/HD.

A century of research on behavior associated with AD/HD has made one thing crystal clear: Many problems can be avoided if early intervention and treatment are provided. Indeed, without early intervention, the impact can be costly and debilitating.

For example, peer rejection in the early years is the greatest predictor of later delinquency, dropping out of school, and mental health problems in adulthood. And an overwhelming majority of youngsters with AD/HD suffer from peer rejection.

In fact, a recent survey of more than five hundred parents at the New York University Child Study Center showed that parents of children with AD/HD reported that their youngsters were nearly three times more likely than typical children to have difficulty getting along with other children in the neighborhood. These children were also more than twice as likely to be picked on and less likely to have many good friends.

Children with untreated AD/HD also are far more likely to be involved in a serious accident, to begin smoking earlier, and to abuse illegal drugs than their typical peers. And, when they grow up, their marriages are many times more likely to experience stress and end in divorce. Worse, it is probable that the prison population is composed of many young and older adults whose AD/HD was undiagnosed and untreated in the early years.

All of this points to the critical need for increased surveillance and action when children are young, as well as avoidance of the tendency among many adults to rationalize away atypical behavior. After all, the implications of this behavior are extreme and costly to the child's future welfare.

AD/HD affects children in all areas of their lives—at home, in school, and in the community—and in a variety of ways.

The Child with AD/HD at Home

Most children with AD/HD are identified as having this disorder because of difficulties they are experiencing in school. Yet, in many instances—and often long before a diagnosis is made— parents harbor suspicions that their child is different from their other children or from other youngsters of the same age.

Seven-year-old Pete's parents, for example, say that calm moments shared with their son have been few and far between. Typically, when Pete is told to do something, his responses have been unpredictable—with even simple requests often resulting in conflict.

From an early age, Pete has habitually gotten into everything—touching breakable items on shelves and taking things out of cabinets, drawers, and the refrigerator without asking. His parents have been reluctant to take Pete out in public and have even felt anxious about inviting friends and family to their home, for fear that Pete would misbehave.

At restaurants, Pete often climbs under and over tables. At the mall, he may run off or cause embarrassing scenes in stores by damaging displays, and in grocery stores, he often plays hide-and-seek.

Getting Pete calmed down for bedtime is often a nightmare for his mom and dad. He fights going to bed and makes repeated "curtain calls" out of his room. When he finally falls asleep, he is all over his bed and often wets his bed as well.

Mealtimes have traditionally been an up-and-down affair for Pete. He can't seem to stay seated and either eats on the move or eats very little. It is not unusual for him to complain about being hungry at bedtime.

At school, Pete's teachers repeatedly report that his work is not up to par and that he has trouble getting along with his peers. When Pete complains that he's dumb and that nobody likes him, his parents try to reassure him. They recognize that he's upset and frustrated. But the truth is, sometimes it's difficult for them to get past their *own* feelings of anguish and frustration.

It takes enormous skill and patience for parents of a child with AD/HD to maintain a positive outlook on the family dynamics. In fact, the best ways for Pete's parents to achieve this goal is to picture the disorder from their son's perspective. His name is called out sternly and repeatedly—to do something, to stop doing something, to pay attention, and so on. All too often he feels well-prepared for a test but gets a poor grade. He longs to take part in group activities at school or in the neighborhood, but no one wants him to be part of their group. And no matter how hard he tries to stay in his seat while doing school work, Pete's teacher is constantly chastising him to stay seated and remain still.

The behavior patterns of children with AD/HD vary from one individual to the next, whether at home, in school, or in other settings. At home, children with AD/HD generally prefer watching television, playing video games, or playing outside. Many have trouble playing independently; thus, when not involved in these preferred activities, they tend to follow a parent around or move from one unsatisfying activity to another. This kind of behavior is likely to frustrate the parent, who in turn is likely to lash out in anger or make unrealistic demands on or threats to the child.

The child with AD/HD shares his parents' frustration. Moreover, when he's yelled at often and loses privileges more often than his siblings do, the effect on his self-esteem can be dramatic. Unfortunately, this, of course, can further frustrate his parents and leave them feeling guilty and incompetent. "What kind of parent am I," the parent often asks, "if I can't even make my child happy?"

A day in the life of a child with AD/HD is also filled with crisis points. Faced with the task of meeting a parent's demands, completing a chore, or making a decision, conflict within himself or with someone else in his environment is generally inevitable. Granted, these crisis points exist with other children as well, but they are far more exaggerated when a child with AD/HD is involved.

When are crises and conflicts most likely to occur at home? During these times:

- Getting out of bed in the morning.
- Getting dressed.
- Eating breakfast.
- Gathering necessary materials/supplies for school.
- Dressing for outdoors.
- Leaving the house on time.
- Waiting for the school bus.
- Changing into after-school clothes.
- Relating events of the school day to a parent.
- Reviewing daily work with a parent.
- Doing homework.
- Preparing the book bag for the next day.
- Playing indoors or outdoors.
- Coming in from outdoors.
- Eating dinner.
- Bathing or showering.
- Preparing for bed.
- Going to and staying in bed.

The Child with AD/HD at School

AD/HD is often misunderstood by teachers and school administrators. Children with the disorder are often labeled troublemakers or slow learners, and their parents are implored to use stronger disciplinary measures or to spend more time with their children studying and doing homework.

This overly simplistic approach only reinforces parents'

feelings of guilt and frustration. In most instances, they have already tried a variety of strategies to help their children be more successful at school.

The child with AD/HD feels equally frustrated and discouraged. She's aware that her name is put on the board more often than are other children's. She knows her grades are not as good as they should be, considering her knowledge of the material. She also recognizes that her peers don't like playing with her because she's impulsive and bossy.

In other words, she feels trapped in a no-win situation. Her teacher is on her back at school; her parents are on her back at home. Yet she may very well be trying as hard as she possibly can to be successful and to meet others' expectations of her.

Many teachers expect that children will finish their seatwork before going out to recess. A wise teacher will recognize that, if three or four days of missed recess fail to modify the child's behavior, the strategy is ineffective. She will then look for other approaches to help improve the child's work habits and behavior in the classroom. After all, a child who is continually punished at school for poor performance or inappropriate behavior—and is then punished at home for the same reasons—will eventually shut down and show little motivation at all to improve.

Bottom line: The school setting is so critical to the child's future success that every effort must be made to soften the negative impact of AD/HD on the child's performance. In Chapter Nine, we have included some very specific strategies for teachers and administrators to better address the challenges presented by children with AD/HD. But suffice it to say that a rigid teacher who, for example, requires that students have both feet flat on the floor when they sit, that the child's bottom belongs firmly planted in the chair, or that neatness counts as much as content on graded papers, will quickly drive the child with AD/HD to despair. Experienced teachers and savvy parents have learned that punitive approaches are not the vehicle to success for the child.

Here are some of the challenges in the classroom that children with AD/HD present most often to their teachers:

- Appears to be bright but does poorly on written assignments.
- Rarely completes written work.
- Often loses his place during class oral reading.
- Copies material incorrectly from the chalkboard or a book.
- Scores inconsistently on tests.
- Seems to daydream a lot.
- Is bossy and impatient with other children.
- Calls out often.
- Is out of seat often to get a drink, go to the bathroom, sharpen a pencil, and so on.
- Often fails to hand in homework (and parents say he did it).
- Has difficulty walking down the hall in line.
- Sits on his legs or works half-standing and half-sitting.

The Child with AD/HD in the Community

Children with AD/HD often show little interest in participating in extracurricular activities that involve groups or teams. The reasons for this stems from their inability to control their impulsiveness, to wait their turn, and to stay focused on such activities. In soccer and baseball games, for example, the child with AD/HD is more likely to be walking the fence, gazing at an airplane flying overhead, or pulling up grass than concentrating on the game.

However, these children often find success in individualized extracurricular activities. In martial arts or dance, for example, where there is more give and take between the child and an instructor, children with AD/HD have an easier time paying attention. These kinds of activities are also less competitive, thus allowing the child more opportunities to experience and enjoy individual success.

When a child with AD/HD goes out to play in the neighborhood, she often comes back soon afterward having had a conflict with "her friend." Often she is rejected by her peers because of her bossiness or unwillingness to follow standard rules of games or those established by the other children. And not surprisingly, she often returns home tearful or angry.

The most important thing for parents, teachers, and members of the community to recognize about AD/HD is that it's an organic problem not unlike asthma, diabetes, or a chronic aching back. Those afflicted with these ailments are victims, just as children who have AD/HD are. And while there may be no cures, there are remedies or treatments for these problems, just as there are for AD/HD.

But in the case of AD/HD, the help and understanding of others is required to provide those remedies. Few children prefer punishment and loss of privileges to rewards and positive attention. Therefore it is crucial to view the child with AD/HD as a victim who longs to perform better, but who simply needs help to do so.

CHAPTER 5

BEHAVIORAL STRATEGIES
FOR THE HOME AND COMMUNITY

*As a second-grader, Margaret made straight A's and B's
and was in the gifted program. Since she entered the
third grade, however, her grades have been slipping.
Her teachers report that she does not pay attention in
class and that much of her work is incomplete. During
work time in the classroom, Margaret is often caught
daydreaming or fidgeting with her pencil. She
daydreams during class discussions as well but always
seems to have the right answer when called upon.*

*At home, Margaret's parents claim that she procrasti-
nates too much. "She'll spend over an hour doing thirty
minutes of homework—unless we provide direct supervision while she is working," says her mother. "And if we
walk away, Margaret's mind appears to wander, or she
starts fidgeting and gets nothing accomplished."*

*Margaret likes to draw and read, but her favorite
activity is playing video games. And while she is able to
sit calmly at the dinner table, she has to be repeatedly
reminded to eat.*

Lately Margaret has been complaining to her parents that she's stupid and that nobody likes her. In response, they mention her previous good grades and try to point out how many birthday parties she's recently been invited to attend. Still, Margaret's parents are concerned about her slipping grades. They also worry that she may be suspended from the gifted program. Above all, they are frustrated because they know how intelligent their daughter is. They watch her complete her assignments perfectly when they sit down with her at night. They are thrilled when they quiz her and she answers nearly all of their questions correctly. What they cannot understand is why, when she gets to school, she appears unable to complete her work or to remember what she's learned the night before.

When they discuss their concern with Margaret's teacher, she assures them that it's "probably just a stage" Margaret is going through. But Margaret's parents don't believe that and make an appointment for their daughter to be evaluated by a child psychologist.

The psychologist spends about thirty minutes with Margaret's parents gathering family, medical, and educational history. This helps to pinpoint potential environmental and medical causes for the symptoms Margaret's parents describe. It also points out patterns of behavior over time. For example, Margaret did well in the unstructured setting of preschool and kindergarten but began having problems in later years, when there were more formal rules for her to follow. The psychologist asks how Margaret behaves in other settings and around different kinds of people.

The psychologist requests copies of all of Margaret's report cards to date. A review of report cards is important in clarifying her academic history and changes over time. The comments teachers have made on Margaret's report cards can also reveal classroom behavior in different grades.

The psychologist asks to look at standardized test score results and samples of Margaret's school work. Finally, he spends time with Margaret discussing her hobbies and interests and who her friends are—trying to get a good general picture of who Margaret is and how she feels about herself.

Margaret's parents make a second appointment for formal testing, including intelligence and achievement tests, projective tests to evaluate personality characteristics, and measures of depression and anxiety. In addition, Margaret's parents are given a checklist to complete based on Margaret's behavior at home. Margaret's teacher is also asked to fill out a checklist regarding behavior she has noticed in the classroom.

When the evaluation process is complete and all of the data are analyzed, the psychologist calls Margaret's parents in for a consultation. Diagnosis: AD/HD. Margaret's parents are not surprised, but they do have many questions to ask the psychologist about how to work with Margaret's teachers, how to tell her siblings about Margaret's disorder, and what strategies they should use to handle Margaret herself.

Parents as Advocates

Nobody knows a child better than her parents. That's why your role in treating your child with AD/HD is so important. Not only must you be well informed about your child's disorder, you must use your knowledge to see that others who care for your child also have a good understanding of what AD/HD is—and isn't. Moreover, you must take whatever steps are necessary to ensure that your child's special needs are being met both inside and outside the home.

It's not an easy job. Caring for a child who has AD/HD can be extremely frustrating. At times you will feel helpless and wonder, "Why me?" But you will also feel hopeful in knowing that you can make a difference in your child's life. As she grows and matures, you *will* notice improvement. And you can take credit for the critical role you played in helping your child be the best she can be.

The first step in becoming an advocate for your child with AD/HD is to learn all you can about her disorder. Reading this book is an excellent start. Also check out the many websites on the Internet devoted to AD/HD. But be cautious, as there is a lot of misinformation about this disorder in cyberspace. Many con artists use the Internet to lure desperate parents to purchase disreputable and unproven services and materials. Your best bet is to log on to a reputable site, such as the one sponsored by the organization ChADD (www.chadd.org), and take advantage of its many useful links. The Centers for Disease Control and Prevention recently named ChADD the National Resource Center on AD/HD. Information to access the Resource Center is available through the website. We also have provided a list of books and other websites on the subject in the Appendix.

Popular magazines often feature articles about AD/HD but, again, beware of extreme and unproven views that are often expressed in these articles. Also, ask your child's doctor to pass along any articles she thinks you might find worthwhile. Professionals in this field have access to many excellent scientific journal articles on AD/HD. Many pharmaceutical companies provide excellent educational materials for parents and children, as well.

Once you have a good working knowledge of AD/HD, your next goal is to find ways to minimize your child's weaknesses and maximize her strengths. Let's start by discussing behavior management strategies that are effective for most children and provide the foundation for modifications you might need to make for your child with AD/HD. (More specific strategies will be discussed later in this chapter.)

A Parent's Toolbox of General Behavior Management Strategies

In an effort to make sure their children with AD/HD follow directions, stay on task, behave in public, and keep up with their school work, many parents admit—often with a great sense of guilt—that they yell a lot or spank their children. Our behavior management approach includes neither of these measures. Rather, it places responsibility on you to teach, model, and reinforce good behavior. It also places responsibility on your child to learn to control his or her behavior.

This approach involves putting several behavior management strategies to work for you and your child:

Determine What Behavior Standards Are Most Important to You

Sit down and make a list, as early as possible in your child's life, of those values and behavior standards that mean the most to you. Then take steps to make sure they will be reinforced by all the adults in your home (such as your spouse, older siblings, or live-in relatives). It's also a good idea to share your standards with your child's daycare staff, baby-sitter, teachers, and even your child's grandparents. That way, everyone is on the same page.

For example, is it important to you for your child to say "Yes, sir" and "Yes, ma'am"? Do you value honesty and respect for other people and property? How important is obedience to you? Whatever pops up on your list, these desirable acts are far more likely to occur if you and other adults in your child's life model these acts *and* if your child is reinforced for exhibiting such behavior.

Make a Habit of Catching Your Child Being Good

Reinforcing good behavior is especially important for a child who has trouble meeting other's expectations on a regular basis. For many adults, however, "catching a child being good" is a difficult habit to develop. That's because there is such a strong tendency to leave a child alone while things are going well and to intervene quickly when behavior goes awry. Yet, both with an individual child and in a group setting with children, paying attention to a child's good behavior has an extremely powerful effect.

Think about it. How would you feel if a friend came to your house and said, "Wow, what a neat kitchen. You sure must be an organized person!" Makes you feel pretty good, doesn't it? On the other hand, what if your friend said, "Wow, I would have a hard time finding anything with all this clutter around. How do you manage?" Not only would you take a big gulp, you'd probably feel pretty knocked down. That's the way it is with kids when all they hear about is what they're doing wrong.

Which statements do you think make a child feel better?

"Thanks for picking up your clothes—your room is sure looking better," OR, *"Your room is always so messy. Get it clean."*

"I like it when you talk in a quiet voice," OR, *"Stop being so loud."*

"It's a lot more fun when you behave so nicely," OR, *"Stop fussing so much and do as you're told."*

Catching children being good comes more naturally for some parents than others, but their children's efforts at behaving well can attest to the success of this approach.

Some frustrated parents of children with AD/HD will say, "My child doesn't do anything right during the day. How can I say something positive when he does nothing good?" This usually means that the parent hasn't been observing carefully enough. Try making a conscious effort for just one day to comment on your child's positive behavior. Also, consider using tangible reinforcers—such as stickers and coupons—which can make this a more positive experience for you and your child. If you watch carefully and you're quick, there will be many actions you can reinforce in this way:

"That's a nice way to sit at the table and eat."

"What a polite way to ask for something."

"You guys are sure using nice voices and playing together well. Keep it up."

"You haven't touched things that aren't yours in a good while. I'm so proud of you!"

Once you see your child's face light up in reaction to your praise and rewards, "catching your child being good" will become habit-forming! And your child will become more aware of his own behavior and increase his efforts to win your praise.

There are other ways to catch your child being good. Try setting up scenarios that guarantee success and allow you to say positive things about a particular kind of behavior that your child exhibits very rarely. For example, suppose you sit down for a meal with the family and, before your child has a chance to begin his usual whining, you say, "I sure do like the way you're sitting so nicely and being polite." Or, for the child who

has trouble staying buckled up in a car seat, buckle him in, give
him a toy to play with, and say, "You look so sweet and safe
playing in your car seat."

Yet another idea: Ask your usually messy child to make up
her bed and pick up her week's dirty clothes from the floor,
then offer to help. As the two of you make progress, comment
on how good the room looks and how such little effort can
make such a huge difference in the appearance of her room.
Don't sermonize or lecture, because it just doesn't work.
Simply express your pleasure and expectations.

Stop and Ask Yourself Some Important Questions

Now that you've established a pretty positive foundation with
your child by modeling good behavior and by reinforcing the
good behavior you want to replace bad behavior, ponder this
fundamental question about children: What is normal and
what is not? When a child is diagnosed with AD/HD, there is
a tendency to attribute all negative behavior to the disorder.
We know that children get into things, say "no," tell lies, take
things that don't belong to them, and avoid doing assigned
tasks. But, in response, do we just stand back and think, "This
too shall pass?" Or do we need to do something about it—and,
if so, what?

Whether we intervene in our child's behavior depends on a
couple of things. First, ask yourself, "Is my child doing any
harm to herself or to any objects?" Second, decide if you, as a
parent, can tolerate your child's behavior. Clearly, for behavior
that is developmentally normal and will disappear with time, it
is far better to ignore the behavior as long as your child will do
no harm to himself, another person, or any object around. So,
safety is an important issue. But another very important issue
is how well you can tolerate the child's behavior. If you are
likely to become more and more angry and frustrated with the

behavior—and you risk eventually losing control of yourself—
then it is best to intervene before you get to this point.

Case in point: If your child is constantly messy, fusses a lot, is
noisy, or has a hard time getting along with others, and in
response, you find yourself quickly at the end of your rope, it is
wise to take some action. Keep in mind that it's harder, at least
initially, to intervene successfully with behavior that you've tolerated in the past and have just now decided to change—for
example, that dirty glass your child puts down wherever she
is; those dirty clothes he lets pile up on the floor; her insis-
tence that you buy her something every time you go into a
store; or his constant talking back to you. The longer your child
has been exhibiting certain behavior (or should we say, the
longer you've put up with it), the harder it will be to change.
That's why you want to start early paying attention and reinforcing good behavior. While AD/HD may stand in the way of
"perfect" behavior, a positive approach toward your child will
minimize many problems.

Learn How to Talk So Your Child Will Listen

Tops on most parents' wish list is the kind of relationship
wherein we talk to our children and they not only listen, but
also do as we ask. It's incredibly frustrating when your child
doesn't respond at all or stubbornly declares, "No, I won't."
Developing a good means of communication involves clearly
stating what you want from your child and having eye contact
with him. In fact, making good eye contact is a valuable life-
time social skill for your child to master. Remember your parents telling you about how important it was to look someone
in the eye when talking or listening to them? It's true! Eye contact is the basis for effective communication, and it will prove
even more important as we proceed in our discussion of other
approaches to guiding your child's behavior and addressing

the more extreme behavior sometimes exhibited by children with AD/HD.

Communicating effectively with your child also involves not repeating yourself over and over again—and with ever-increasing volume and intensity. Indeed, it's easy for your child to learn to ignore you until telltale signs appear—your face grows red, the sound of exasperation creeps into your voice, or you begin issuing threats.

You really don't want to get to that point. It's simply not good for your health, nor will it help keep your special relationship with your child healthy. So, start early and get into the habit of communicating with your child at an early age. That way, you avoid at least some of the power struggles that come with being a parent.

Be a Smart Parent

Kids love to explore. Doors, cabinets, high places, and barricades often seem to flash an invisible message that screams to children's ears: "Check me out!" Matches, lighters, and knives are intriguing long before a child can understand their potential dangers. The good news is, many potentially undesirable actions can be avoided with a little parental foresight. For example, do you dress your three-year-old in a beautiful outfit and then serve tomato soup for lunch? Do you leave matches or car keys around a child who likes to take things and hide them? Prevention includes such things as childproofing a room by putting fragile or hazardous objects out of your child's reach, installing cabinet and drawer locks, and keeping doors closed to rooms that are off-limits or that lead to the outside, as well as not taking your child along to places where his behavior might be disruptive. After all, avoiding situations in which your child is likely to be out of control is just being a smart parent. It saves you a lot of stress and doesn't penalize your child for behavior he might be unable to control.

Yet another form of prevention involves preparing your child for new experiences. Here's an example: Most children go to the movies for the first time at about two to four years of age. Let's follow a young child through this maiden voyage. You walk with him into the lobby of the theater, and there sits the concession stand. Your child immediately starts asking for all kinds of goodies, and your mind begins mentally checking the family budget to see what you can afford. You almost miss the start of the movie because of the lengthy push and pull to get your child to forgo the chewy dinosaurs and choco-balls for a soft drink and a tub of buttered popcorn.

Next, you enter the theater itself. You've been there lots of times and take it in stride. What your child sees, however, is an enormous dark space with the largest TV screen he's ever seen up in front. Naturally, given all these factors, his tendency is to get pretty excited—or scared—and ask lots of questions. You, however, expect him to be very quiet and still. BIG CONFLICT.

How can we limit these kinds of conflicts? By preparing our children in advance—not only by talking about where we're taking them, but by making our behavior expectations clear. Example: "We're going to Nanna and Grandpa's house in a little while. Remember how important it is that you're polite and talk quietly. We'll be real proud of you."

Any parent who has taken a child along to the grocery store knows what a challenge this can be. After all, there are aisles filled with wonderful products targeted at kids, all those nice tall displays, and so much activity. Also, grocery trips often occur late in the day when everyone is tired and cranky. Wise parents use preventive strategies—such as bringing along a book or little game or toy to keep the child busy during the shopping trip. Some parents use a strategy called redirection— that is, when your child begins to engage in an inappropriate behavior, you redirect her to a different behavior. For example, while in the supermarket, you might have your child help put the groceries in the cart after you have taken them off the shelf. Or, you might count with her how many shopping carts you pass. At home, redirection might entail giving your child her favorite toy or a cracker to chew on to direct her away from the stereo dials, or asking your child to get more milk from the refrigerator to keep him from picking on his sister.

Keep Cool

With all these approaches, self-control on your part is important. Many of the most frustrating actions—the spilled cup of milk caused by reaching across the table, the toys left all over the floor, and the loud playing—are typical behavior of young children. But, even with your older child, if you get bent out of shape over these incidents, your child won't learn to distinguish between your response to something he did without thought and something that is harmful or clearly out of bounds. Also, if you're walking around on edge all the time, where's the fun in being a parent? And it should be fun and satisfying most of the time.

Master the Contingency Approach

Children of all ages have favorite activities—things they look forward to daily. These might include watching a favorite television program, riding their bicycle, playing a computer game, calling a friend or grandparent, or borrowing the car. The contingency approach uses a simple formula: Before your child can do what she *wants* to do, she must do what she *needs* to do or what you want her to do. Here are some examples of how this approach can be used with children of different ages:

> *"Jonathon, if you want to watch your video, you have to eat six more bites of vegetables and finish your hamburger."*

"Susie, you can go outside and ride your bike as soon as your room is cleaned up."

"Arthur, if you sit quietly in the cart while we're at the grocery store, we'll stop and get some ice cream on the way home."

"Sherry, if you want to go skating with your friends tonight, you have to get your term paper finished first."

"Alex, if you want to use the car to go to the mall, you must apologize to your sister for fighting with her and show that you can treat her nicely."

This simple but powerful approach can be used with children as young as twelve to eighteen months of age. And to make it work, you need only follow a few important steps. First, you must be able to identify the things that your child likes to do most. Often youngsters will help you do this by making suggestions about things they like to do. However, you must also be aware of activities they are looking forward to in the near future. That way, you can use these as incentives as well.

Second, the activities your child wants to take part in must be timed appropriately. In other words, you can't talk about an outing to the park on Saturday as an incentive if it's only Tuesday. In fact, as a rule of thumb, try not to use an activity as an incentive if it is scheduled more than an hour or two away. In addition, the incentive should not be elaborate or extraordinary. Those things your child looks forward to regularly are the most desirable incentives to use.

Third, avoid using as a consequence an activity *you're* looking forward to as much as—or more than—your child. Suppose you've been counting on having dinner at a new restaurant in town, and your child knows how much you're looking forward to it. Saying to him, "We won't be going out to eat tonight if you don't clean up your room," won't work. On the contrary, it places the child in the position of being able to sabotage or control what *you* want to do rather than your controlling what *he* is supposed to do.

Fourth, and most important, be consistent in following through on what you say. Do *not* change rules after you have made them. If you want your child to finish her homework before she goes outside, your job is to make sure that the homework is done before she walks out the door. There is no need for further negotiation or debate. The criterion is clear: Either the homework is complete or it isn't.

Finally, you must be willing to tolerate your child's not doing what you want him to do while ensuring that he does not get the promised reward. With children who are extremely resistant to following directions, use the contingency approach at every opportunity. Consistency in using this approach—even for simple directions—helps a child learn that he must listen to what you say. Therefore, you can use even simple contingencies, such as the following:

> *"Malcolm, please put this glass on the table for me before I put the video in for you."*

> *"Carlie, please put the pillow back on the couch and then I will get you a drink."*

Later, as your child's efforts to follow instructions improve, you can reserve the contingency approach for those tasks that create the greatest stress.

Stick to Your Guns

When children lose rewards, they may respond, "I didn't want to do that anyway." This is typical and is aimed at getting you to give in. Don't do it. Be strong and know that the privilege or activity you've taken away probably is important to your child. And even if it means that homework doesn't get done for a few days or a room doesn't get cleaned up for a week, your youngster will eventually give in and show you that the reward was an important one after all. From your perspective, it's a matter of being willing to lose a few battles in order to win the war.

In other words, if you tell your child that she's not going outside until she's cleaned up her toys, stick to it. Remind your child that you'd love for her to have a chance to go outside. Then remind yourself that you're not the bad guy. *She's* the one who is preventing it from happening by not taking responsibility and picking up her toys. There's no need to raise your voice and no need to get bent out of shape. Be nice and objective about it.

Occasionally, this approach fails—and here's why. First, your child may have learned that "reverse psychology" works with you. In other words, if she acts as if it doesn't matter, you'll throw up your arms in frustration and give in. But even if it appears not to matter to her, hang in there for at least a few days and follow through on what you said you would do. Chances are, you'll quickly discover that it matters a lot to her.

Another reason this approach may not work is that you've misread what is important to your child. If your motivator isn't motivating, your child might not be encouraged to do what you want her to do or what she needs to do.

Your child may even sabotage the process on purpose. Let's say you tell him, "You can go outside as soon as you finish your homework." In response, your child mutters to himself, "Well, it's hot outside and nasty Billy will be out there to pick on me again. I'd rather stay in here anyway." In this instance, while you may have chosen a contingency that typically motivates your child, there are better reasons for him *not* to earn the reward this time.

Finally, keep in mind that as much as she wants the reward, a child with AD/HD may not be able to complete a required task. But this approach, used over the course of several days, will help you determine what is within—or beyond—your child's control.

Send Your Child the Right Message

When disciplining your child with AD/HD, it's important to remember that the message you send should be that you love *him* but don't like his *behavior*. Granted, many of us feel compelled to explain to our children all of the intricacies of why we do things a certain way. But this strategy appears to do little good and, in fact, may even harm children with AD/HD. Very often, they will try to take advantage of your willingness to discuss disciplinary measures in an effort to manipulate the situation. It's their way of delaying meeting their responsibilities. It's also a way for them to control the situation.

You should recognize, however, that this type of behavior often results from a child's perceived inability to perform a task easily. That is, she recognizes that she has great difficulty sustaining her attention—say, on homework—for a long period of time, and it becomes very difficult and unpleasant for her. Likewise, she may recognize that she doesn't have the persistence to get her room cleaned up and is destined for failure if she is asked to do so. Consequently, her tendency is to battle against this kind of structure.

Nevertheless, your providing consistency, realistic and reasonable expectations, and support and reassurance, should soon result in greater success for her.

Try the Restriction Approach

Think of this strategy as a variation of the contingency approach. With restriction, a valued activity or privilege is taken away, usually for misbehavior or as a result of the child's not doing what is expected. So, fighting with a sibling might mean TV restriction, talking back might mean outdoor restriction, and misbehaving at the dinner table might mean restriction from having a friend over on the weekend. But beware of one common mistake parents make when using restrictions: Avoid putting your child on restriction for more than one day at a time.

For example, Ben's parents recently put him on telephone and computer restriction for one week for not telling the truth. The very next day, he told another lie—which presented a dilemma for his parents. Should they add another week of restriction, or should they take away something else? If they add time, it becomes an even less meaningful consequence. If they take away something else, Ben soon may have nothing left to take.

Let's suppose that the next day, Ben told no lies. Nor did he on the following day. When he asks if he can use the phone or computer, he is told that he has five days left on restriction. So, where's the incentive? The idea is to keep as much leverage available to you as you possibly can. When you take toys away for three weeks because your child is destructive with them, you have given up the toys as leverage for that period of time to help teach improved behavior. In fact, you're practically guaranteed quicker and more efficient results when you say, "You can have your toys back when you're ready to play nicely with them," or, "Your toys will be put away for the rest of the day, and we'll take them out in the morning and see if you can play with them nicely." That's because this approach not only communicates clear expectations and consequences, but also gives your child an opportunity to do better.

Are contingencies and restrictions useful approaches for teaching responsibility? You bet! But not every task or kind of behavior should require applying these approaches. The hope is that, as time passes, your child with AD/HD will try harder to do the right thing independently—or, at the very least, will respond to subtle verbal prompts or reminders.

Turn to Time-out

Sometimes a child's behavior becomes so disruptive—or you begin to feel so frustrated or angry—that the best approach is to remove him from the situation. The object of *time-out* is to deprive the child of attention or positive reinforcement. Sitting your child in the corner, however, rarely works, since he need only make noise, rock back and forth, or stand up to get your attention. Moreover, this strategy is likely to encourage the continuation of his unacceptable behavior. Thus, the best location for time-out at home is in your child's room. As with the contingency approach, several principles should be followed.

For starters, before sending your child to his room, follow this three-step approach. First, tell him clearly the kind of behavior you expect him to display or to cease displaying. Some examples:

"Brian, sit on the sofa quietly."

"Erin, stop fighting with Cynthia."

"Mark, go sit down at the table now and get started with your homework."

If he doesn't comply, state the action you want (or don't want) again and indicate the consequences. Examples:

"Tonya, leave the knobs on the stereo alone or you will go sit in your room."

"Eric, set the table now or you won't be able to watch America's Funniest Home Videos *later tonight."*

"Sally, clean up the mess you made on the kitchen table or you can't go outside and play with your friends."

Of course, while it's nice to phrase *all* statements in positive terms, a "stop-doing" statement is typically the first thing that comes to mind when a child is obviously not listening. And that's fine, since these approaches should help reduce the number of negative statements you make.

Finally, if your child persists, send him to his room with these instructions: "Stay in your room until you are ready to _____." Essentially, this approach makes the *child* responsible for deciding when he is ready to comply, and at that point he can come out of his room.

When using time-out, avoid telling your child to go to his room and think about what he did. Instead, focus on the behavior that you'd like to see rather than what you saw. That way, when the child is in his room, instead of moping about what he's already done, he too can focus on the kind of behavior it will take for him to be able to leave the room. He can also then monitor whether he is ready to exhibit the kind of behavior you've requested or not.

What to do if your child comes out of his room and continues to display the same disruptive behavior? Send him back to his room again with the reminder that he can come out again when he is ready to behave the way you requested. This should be the last chance you give him to change his behavior voluntarily. Should he be sent back to his room again, *you* then decide when he is ready to come out. Your child loses the privilege of deciding when he is ready to come out of his room.

Again, make it clear to your child that you love *him* but that his *behavior* needs to change. Your message must be that you want to be with him but that first he must behave well—and he will have to stay in his room until he is ready to make that decision.

What about children who refuse to stay in their rooms? In instances like these, a child recognizes that she can still control the situation by coming and going—and getting attention from you for that. The following strategy may appear quite extreme; nevertheless, it meets the criteria for a very sound behavior management program. It is not punitive; rather, it results in an improvement of a child's behavior, and the child has control over administration of the consequences.

Here is how the approach works: Reverse the doorknobs on your child's bedroom door so that the locking mechanism is on the outside. Then, after she comes out of her room for the second time and continues to display the same disruptive behavior, you can send her back to her room and lock the door. Repeat your instructions: "You may come out as soon as you are ready to _____ ."

Once your child is back in her room for the third time and realizes that the door is locked, she may scream and bang or kick the door. Try to ignore this temper tantrum. You may also need to childproof her room as much as possible before using this procedure by removing any objects that might be breakable or harmful. But, again, do not allow your child out of her room until she is ready to behave the way you want her to.

Thirty seconds after initially locking the door, feel free to go back and ask if she's ready to come out and do as you requested. If she is not ready, walk away and return in another minute and a half. Then repeat this process about every five minutes thereafter. Once she is ready to come out of her room, deal only with the behavior you requested of her previously. If she doesn't comply, send her back to her room and wait a little longer before checking to see if she is ready to come back out again.

When you first begin using this approach, your child may spend a good part of the first few days in her room. However, once she realizes that she is not in control of the situation—and that you will be consistent—even the behavior of a child with AD/HD should improve.

Remember, harsh as this seems, it is not an inhumane approach. Granted, it may be difficult for you to continue the process, but your consistency is the key to the success of this method. Keep in mind throughout the ordeal that your child makes the choice of when she is ready to come out of the room, and that her choice is based on a desire to behave in an appropriate way.

Time-out can also be used effectively in public. At restaurants, at malls, and in supermarkets, children who are easily overstimulated generally demonstrate some of their worst behavior. The use of contingencies in these situations may be effective and should always be tried first. In fact, unless you've exhausted every other approach discussed thus far—or you're feeling frustrated and overwhelmed—you should always save packing everyone in the car and heading back home as a last resort. That's because leaving the scene only reinforces your child's feelings of being able to control the situation and call the shots.

A better way to deal with inappropriate behavior in public? Try taking your child into a bathroom or a hallway and indicating that you will stay there until she is ready to behave. The unstimulating environment of a restaurant bathroom might be all the encouragement a child needs to straighten up once she realizes that you are serious about your willingness to stay there as long as necessary. Realistically, this won't work if you're the only adult there with several children. And if that's the case, you just might need to avoid these situations, if possible, and concentrate on establishing control at home first.

In sum, time-out is an effective strategy for a number of reasons. First, because it separates you and your child; it allows you to cool off and not get angry and frustrated. It also removes your child from a reinforcing environment. Second, time-out places your child in charge of deciding when she is ready to improve her behavior. Third, and best of all, time-out provides an opportunity to de-escalate situations that can easily get out of hand.

To make it work, however, you must intervene when your child first begins to behave inappropriately. If you wait until the behavior gets out of hand, it will be much more difficult to bring the situation under control.

Both the contingency and time-out approaches should be used consistently. They help children structure their own behavior and provide much-needed relief for parents who feel as if they are constantly on their children's backs. Also, since they can be equally effective with children without AD/HD, these strategies can be used to instill acceptable behavior in *all* your children. That way, the child with AD/HD doesn't feel as if he is being singled out.

Consider Creating Chore Charts

For children with AD/HD who are ages five and up, various types of charts can prove to be valuable assets in molding and reinforcing positive behavior. What's more, when charts are tied to valued consequences, many children actually enjoy— and often benefit from—having this visual reminder.

To make a chore chart, sit down with your child and choose no more than three actions or tasks that she must accomplish before receiving certain privileges. These may include such goals as cleaning up her room, playing nicely with her sister, completing her homework, reading for thirty minutes, sitting quietly at the table, taking out the trash with just one reminder, or being ready when the school bus arrives. Next, make a list of privileges—or things your child likes to do. Then decide how many goals she must meet to earn these privileges. If she completes two out of three tasks, she may earn all but her most valued privilege (watching television, for example). If she does not accomplish any of the goals within a given day, she forfeits all privileges, and, in addition, may have to go to bed thirty minutes early.

Whenever possible—or at least initially—consequences should be administered the same day. Later, weekly consequences can also be used, based on how many checks or stars the child has earned by week's end.

Suppose your son is given an opportunity to earn three checks in a day, or a total of fifteen during the five-day school week. If he is looking forward to seeing a movie with friends on Friday evening or going to a skating party on Saturday, he may have to earn at least twelve checks during the week to enjoy that privilege. Once a child has developed a pattern of responsibility and can accomplish these tasks without fuss and constant reminders, you can substitute new goals for old ones (or even discontinue the chart altogether).

Be sure, however, to change the menu of consequences as your child's interests change. While it's not unusual for a youngster to say, "I didn't want to watch television anyway!" it's important that you remain persistent and tolerate some failures for a few days while working toward the larger goals of improved behavior and performance. For instance, if your child decides that he can live without television for a few days, add some other privilege to the consequences that he can earn along with television time. That way, it shouldn't take long before the chart is doing the work for you, and your child becomes more responsible and easier to manage.

On page 88, you will find an example of a chore chart, which uses money as the incentive. This approach works well for children who enjoy buying certain things (CDs, doll accessories, or skateboard posters, for example) and who respond to the daily accumulation of earnings and a weekly payoff.

Charts also provide you with opportunities to reinforce the pride you are taking in your child's good behavior. In other words, be ready for plenty of opportunities to catch your child being good!

Setting Up the Child with AD/HD for Success at Home

Now that we have provided you with a general foundation for behavior management, here are some more specific approaches

DAILY CHORE CHART

Martin, Age 8   Week of: _____

DAY	CLEANS UP ROOM	READY FOR SCHOOL ON TIME	FEEDS DOG (1 reminder only)	BONUS	TOTAL
Monday	☆	☆	☆	Took out trash. +25¢	$ 1.00
Tuesday	Threw everything under bed!	☆	☆		.50
Wednesday	☆	☆	3 reminders and still not done.	Went to bed quickly, no fuss. +25¢	.75
Thursday	☆	Argued over sneakers or shoes.	☆		.50
Friday	☆	☆	Overnight visit with friends.	Took out trash. +25¢	.75 Payoff
Saturday	☆		☆	Helped vacuum and dust. 25¢	.75
Sunday	☆		☆	Washed car. Picked up pine cones and pulled weeds.	.75

that will make family and home life more pleasant for you and your child with AD/HD.

Give Your Child a Simple but Straightforward Explanation of What AD/HD Is and Help Her to Understand How the Disorder Affects Her

Children under six years of age are not likely to understand big words like "Attention Deficit/Hyperactivity Disorder." So, explain to them in simple terms what's happening in their brain to make them act differently. If you have trouble finding the right words to explain AD/HD, there are several good children's books you can read to your child or give to her to read (see Appendix). If your youngster is old enough to read one of these books alone, however, be sure to discuss the material she's read and answer all of her questions afterward.

It's a good idea to have other siblings read or listen to the material and participate in discussions as well. They can serve as allies and supporters for the child's efforts. Also, if they have a clear understanding of AD/HD, they will be less likely to make fun of efforts that fall short of success.

Let Him Know He's Not Alone

Tell him how many children struggle with AD/HD, and make sure he knows that you, his siblings, his teachers, and other caregivers and professionals are "on his team."

Explain Your Child's Problem to Other Family Members

Then point out and explain why sometimes her behavior must be treated differently from theirs.

Make a List of Family Rules and Review Them with All Your Children

Make sure each one is understood, and then post them on the refrigerator as a reminder. The best time to establish rules is immediately following conflicts and dilemmas. For example, suppose your children are getting up from the table repeatedly during meals and are interfering with your desire to have everyone sit at the table to enjoy a quiet meal together. In response, you might introduce a rule such as Rule 5 in the example below about asking to be excused before leaving the table. Rules can also be introduced to family members by saying, "Maybe we should have a rule for that," or, "Why don't we think of a rule we can set up to help us with this problem?" Whenever possible, involve your children in helping to establish the rules and always discuss new rules before implementing them.

Family Rules

1. We pick up after ourselves.
2. We talk politely to one another.
3. We do our chores every day.
4. We don't interrupt.
5. We ask to be excused before leaving the table.
6. We do our work before we play.
7. We let someone know where we are at all times.

Assign Your Youngster with AD/HD Chores She Can Handle Easily and Set Up a Reward System for Completing Each Task

For example, you might place stickers or stars on a chart and agree that a completely filled row can be cashed in for a special treat. When first introducing this approach, however, give lesser rewards for having just a few stickers, as this will not only help your children get used to this system, but should also motivate them.

Gradually Add More Difficult Chores to a Child's List As She Masters the Easier Ones

This will help her develop a sense of responsibility. Also, if she is challenged and prevails, her self-esteem will soar. On the flip side, if she fails, be sure to reduce the number and difficulty of chores to make success more probable.

Whenever Possible, Let Your Child with AD/HD Set Her Own Personal Goals, Then Work at Her Own Pace at Achieving Them

That way, she can experience the joy of accomplishing something on her own—and this can be extremely motivating.

Once Goals Are Set, Work Up Parent-Child Contracts

Discuss each goal, then write and sign a contract, with each of you outlining what action you plan to ensure that the goal is met. Suppose your child's goal is to clean her room twice a week. She would write, "I will clean my room twice a week," then sign her name. Next, you would write a similar statement below hers—something like, "I will help her reach this goal by reminding her of it on Thursdays and Sundays. When she has cleaned her room as promised for two consecutive weeks, we will go to see a movie together." Should this approach not work for several consecutive weeks, it might be necessary to return to looking at shorter-term goals that can be rewarded immediately.

Make Sure the Expectations You Have of Your Child with AD/HD Are Realistic and that the Consequences for Poor or No Performance Are Realistic

Let's return to Margaret's case, described at the beginning of this chapter. Margaret's mom expected that her daughter would be able to finish her homework in a short period of time—and unsupervised—and that she would receive all A's on her report card. But short-term expectations like these are setting Margaret up for failure (although this might be a long-term goal to work toward). Similarly, depriving Margaret of her favorite activities—such as drawing, reading, and video games—because of lack of success only leads to a more frustrated child and strips her of the few things she consistently does well and enjoys. In other words, expectations should be such that your children are able to attain success often enough to earn rewards and feel good about their accomplishments.

Point Out How Your Child's Actions Affect What Happens Around Her

Suppose, for example, that your child starts hitting the dog for tearing up her favorite doll—the very one you told her to put away many times in the past thirty minutes. Only when you review with your children how what they do (or don't do) affects what happens afterward do they begin to become accountable for the consequences of their actions.

Help Your Child Find an Activity in Which She Can Excel

Children with AD/HD often suffer from poor self-esteem and constantly think, "I'm no good at anything." This is particularly true for children with siblings who shine at certain activities. To boost your child's self-esteem, help her find activities in which she cannot easily be compared to other family members or to her circle of friends, as well as ones that do not involve groups of youngsters competing against one another. These might include such activities as knitting, putting puzzles together, playing an unusual musical instrument (such as the harmonica), martial arts, or horseback riding.

Give Instructions for Tasks One at a Time

Children with AD/HD often cannot handle multiple commands and are confused by the use of complex language. Therefore, use simple and direct language, providing instructions for one task at a time until your child shows that she is capable of processing more than one step. In addition, preface your instructions with your child's name, as in, "Marie, put your plate in the sink, please." When you use this approach, a child is more likely to pay attention and absorb what you are saying.

When Giving Oral Instructions to a Child with AD/HD, Maintain Constant Eye Contact with Her

That way, you can ensure she is listening. If you have your doubts, ask her to repeat your instructions aloud.

Give Instructions in Statement Form

Many parents make the mistake of asking, "Are you ready to go to bed?" when what they really mean is, "It's time to go to bed." When you ask a question, your child may assume that you are willing to accept whatever answer you receive. And, while there are times when you certainly want to give your child choices, be sure not to mistakenly provide options when you do not mean to do so.

Encourage Your Children to Write Daily "To-Do" Lists for Themselves

This helps for two reasons. First, it helps your child get organized. Second, checking off items she has completed will give her a strong sense of accomplishment. Using a marker board can be helpful for maintaining current lists of things to do and upgrading lists easily.

When a Child Appears Unmotivated to Complete Tasks, Use the Contingency Approach

Remember, it works like this: "If you want to do such and such [have a friend spend the night, for example], you must do such and such first."

Keep in Mind that Children with AD/HD Need Regular Routines

Establish firm bedtimes, wake-up times, and study hours—and stick to them!

When Angry, Try to Avoid Yelling and Punishing Your Child

Instead, use time-out to help alleviate your—and her—feelings of frustration.

Make It Clear to Your Child that the Focus Is on His Behavior

You can best do this by constantly reinforcing that you love *him*. What you don't like is his *behavior.*

Give Your Children Choices

Let them decide whether they want to demonstrate the correct behavior or deal with the consequences if they choose not to cooperate. That way, youngsters learn to make responsible decisions.

Deal Promptly with Inappropriate Behavior

For example, if your child is touching something she shouldn't be touching, playing at the table with her food, throwing things around the house, or fighting with another child, you must intervene promptly rather than letting the behavior persist or escalate until you are frustrated and angry.

Ignore Behavior that Is Not Dangerous and Is Not Interfering with What Your Child Should Be Doing

If your child is slumped in her chair while doing her homework, for instance, ignore her posture so long as she continues to work. In other words, if you pounce on every little thing, you will generate more conflict than you resolve.

Make Special Efforts to Let Your Child Know When She Is Behaving or Performing Well

Some parents of children with AD/HD complain that it's difficult to find anything that their child does do right. What this often means is that the parents have stopped looking. Whether it's helping out around the house, politely answering the telephone, or greeting a neighbor, there are many opportunities to give credit where credit is due.

Keep Caregivers Consistent

Once parents of children with AD/HD find behavior strategies that work at home, these should also be used by a child's other caregivers. Otherwise, the child will be confused, and the goal of her being responsible for her own behavior will not be met.

Unfortunately, when grandparents are intent on being permissive—or when a noncustodial parent is unwilling to follow the plan—there are likely to be setbacks. In such circumstances, however, continued structure at home will help your child learn that the rules are always the same there, even though they may change elsewhere. The hope is that eventually your child will generalize what he gets at home and school to other settings.

Help Your Child Learn to Monitor Her Own Behavior

By using such phrases as "boss yourself" or "check yourself out," you cue your child that better self-control is needed at that time. When used consistently, this approach helps your child become more aware of her behavior and begin to assert greater control over herself. With academic tasks, for example, help train your child to "check in with herself" at frequent intervals to evaluate if she has understood what she has just read, if she is making progress on her worksheet, if she is copying the sentences correctly, and so forth. Using this strategy, a child may learn to stop after each sentence she reads to be sure she understands it before moving on. And this will help prevent her from getting to the bottom of the page and realizing she doesn't remember what she has read—a common problem for children with AD/HD.

Challenge Your Child to Motivate Herself

Teach her to come up with ways to work faster or more efficiently. For example, if she got three questions correct on one
reading comprehension passage, challenge her to answer four
questions correctly the next time. Set a timer to see how long
it takes her to complete a long division problem, then challenge her to do the next one in a little less time. If she needs to
meet certain criteria for performance—such as completing a
task within a certain period of time or a certain level of correct
responses—help her to develop these. Have her think of
and write down what she wants to do when she finishes her
work. Be careful, though, to use this approach to generate
greater success rather than greater failure. By setting up a
model that spurs motivation, the child can then start setting up
her own challenges and incentives to work more quickly and
more efficiently.

Home Behavior Management
to Support Success at School

Many parents mistakenly believe that what happens to their
children with AD/HD in school is beyond their control. On the
contrary, you can play a major role in setting your child up for
success in this arena as well.

Again, your role as advocate comes into play. Talking to and
educating your child's school administrators and teachers
about the special needs of your youngster with AD/HD is crucial, as is your willingness to help them find ways to help your
child shine. Granted, this can be exhausting at times, but the
fact is that success at school for a child with AD/HD very often
hinges on whether he has a parent willing to go to bat for him.

There also are steps you can take at home to set your
child up for success at school. Here are some tried-and-true
guidelines:

Establish a Routine for What Happens When Your Child Arrives Home from School

A good start is to ask, "What's the best thing that happened at school today?" This helps a child think of school in positive terms. After that, the routine may include a snack, changing clothes, and sitting down to homework. Try not to vary the routine from day to day, however. Remember, children with AD/HD thrive on structure and routine, so keeping things the same will save battles, negotiations, and unnecessary arguments about when to do homework and study.

Provide a Quiet Place Free from Distractions Where Your Child Can Do Homework and Study

Some children respond better working in the same place every day. Others need a change of scenery to stay motivated and focused. In any case, always try a study setting for several days before concluding that it doesn't fill the bill for your child.

What do you do if your child insists on studying while the radio or stereo is playing? Actually, some children with AD/HD do better with quiet music playing in the room. That's because it helps to drown out other sounds inside and outside the house that might otherwise be distracting. Often, it's trial and error finding the correct setting and best conditions under which your child can work most efficiently. What's more, these may change with age and the challenge of certain tasks. But as a rule of thumb, your child will complete his work faster, more easily, and more efficiently in a quiet setting if you have established a sound routine.

Use a Study or Office Setting for Homework and Studying

Your goal should be to get your child in the habit of working in a work setting. Kitchen tables, sofas, and the floor may be comfortable locations, but they are also generally high-traffic areas and do not send the message, "This is serious work that needs to be completed to the best of your abilities." On the other hand, after trying various settings and positions, you might find that your child fares better doing work standing up or lying across the bed. While it may make you a bit uncomfortable giving the green light to these habits, give it a try if that's what your child wants. Just make sure he understands that he must prove that he benefits from this alternative setting.

Check Your Child's Book Bag Daily and Help Him Get Organized

Parents of children with AD/HD who check backpacks infrequently often find notes, reminders, flyers, and graded papers days or weeks old. If you make this part of your daily routine, your child is less likely to be penalized for missing important deadlines. Also, if you begin this practice at an early age, your high-school student will be less resistant to your going through his book bag.

Use a Daily Homework Assignment Sheet That the Teacher Initials Daily

Younger children with AD/HD have real trouble remembering to write down their homework assignments. Or they may hurriedly scribble them down, then not be able to read their own handwriting later. A better idea? Have the teacher check and initial that homework assignments are recorded correctly. This will make it easier for your child to complete the correct and required work at home.

Keep in mind, though, that if you make your child responsible for getting her teacher to sign this sheet, this strategy may not work. After all, if she could remember to take the sheet to her teacher each day, she probably also would remember to write down her assignments. Moreover, since teachers may get particularly busy toward the end of the day or class period, it's helpful to have alternative plans in place. One idea is to have a buddy in class check to be sure your child's homework is written down correctly. Another is to keep the phone numbers of a few children in the class who can be called to verify assignments if there are any questions about them.

Review Your Child's Homework Assignments Nightly to Make Sure She Has Completed All of Them

Getting your child used to this routine at a young age avoids conflicts later as your child hits adolescence. The purpose of the check is not to make sure all answers are correct, but to be sure that the assignment is complete and done neatly. You should also take this opportunity to praise your child for good effort and to make suggestions for improvement for the next day. What do you do if there's a problem with the assignment? Maybe it's messy, or perhaps it's incomplete. If so, fall back on the contingency approach. Tell your child, "You need to do this part over before you get to watch TV [or read or go outside or get on the computer]."

Limit Homework to a Reasonable Amount of Time

Some parents complain that they are up working with their elementary school children until ten or eleven o'clock at night on a regular basis doing homework. Home life should not be totally consumed with school-related matters—either for the child or the parent. In fact, when this occurs repeatedly, working parents come to dread the end of the workday and heading home, while stay-at-home parents dread the sound of the school bus stopping outside at the end of the day. And with good reason: The battles are ready to begin!

By a reasonable amount of homework time, what do we mean? No more than two to two and one-half times the amount of time that primary-grade children are expected to spend on homework and no more than 50 percent more than the amount of time middle- and high-school students are expected to spend on homework. For example, if a third-grader's homework is expected to take about twenty minutes, your child with AD/HD should not have to spend more than forty to fifty minutes on that assignment. Similarly, if a tenth-grader has about an hour's worth of homework and studying, he should not spend more than one-and-a-half hours on that work. You may need to consult your child's teachers to find out how long they estimate students should spend on homework each day.

To help your child complete his homework more quickly within this reasonable amount of time, using a timer and allowing periodic breaks can be beneficial. Set the timer initially for five to ten minutes and encourage your child to work hard on the material until the bell rings. The timer should be sitting on your child's desk or table so that she has a visual reminder of the need to move along. When the bell rings, return to check over your child's work and progress. If she has done well, she can take a break for a few minutes. Then set the timer for two to three minutes longer than during the previous session and repeat the same procedure.

The purpose of this process is to get your child used to working independently and for longer and longer periods of time without a break or assistance. Nevertheless, be available to assist when necessary. Should your child not complete the assignment in the allotted time, the books should get put away anyway. You can then write a note to the teacher indicating how long your child worked on her homework and that she will work harder the next day to try to complete the whole assignment. Also, let your child know that she doesn't get to enjoy any recreational activities for the remainder of that day, since she has not yet completed that day's homework. That means no TV, no CD player or stereo, no phone time, no computer, no outdoor play, and so forth. The next day begins with a clean slate and, one hopes, increased efforts to complete homework.

Number Your Child's Assignments and Worksheets or Give Them to Her One at a Time, So She Doesn't Feel Overwhelmed

Many children with AD/HD have a tendency to spend as much time shuffling papers around as they do trying to complete their assignments. Or they waste a lot of time trying to figure out where to start. Numbering the order of homework assignments or giving them to her one by one may help your child to become more organized and efficient—or at least get the work done more quickly. Keep in mind, too, that your child's workspace should be clutter-free, except for the paper she is working on. Too many books and papers in the area easily distract some children.

Find Extra Help to Assist Your Child with a Particularly Weak Subject

Many parents feel overwhelmed themselves by the new material children are learning today and unqualified to assist their child. The simplest approach is to use an older sibling or classmate to help your child, but private tutors are also available in most areas and usually offer the benefit of teacher training. Check at your child's school for a list of teachers and other adults who are interested in tutoring. Local high-school and college students might also be interested in helping your child. In addition, there are many commercial tutoring firms that do a good job of motivating children and pinpointing strengths and weaknesses in their learning and work habits. Many of these businesses have special training and experience working with children with AD/HD.

Whomever you hire, the more recommendations you can get in advance through other parents and friends, or by attending PTA or local ChADD meetings, the greater the likelihood that your child and the tutor will work well together and that the tutoring will be beneficial. Using a tutor also takes some of the pressure off you, and that should diminish stress levels at home.

Make Yourself Available to Work with Your Child's Teacher When Your Youngster Needs Extra Help

When you are unhappy with the quality of work coming home, when the teacher sends home many notes about your child's poor performance in school, or when you have other concerns about your youngster's work or behavior, it's wise to act quickly. Sitting around for weeks waiting for your child's report card or waiting for the teacher to suggest a conference may compound the problems, and your child's self-esteem suffers. Request a meeting with your child's teacher to talk about how all the parties involved can help your youngster be more successful. (Check Chapter Seven for more resources.)

Dealing with *Your* Feelings

Parents of children with AD/HD, particularly mothers, often report feeling "torn"—totally dejected and ineffective in controlling their child on the one hand and extremely guilty about the anger they feel toward the child on the other. Many often question whether they really love their child, considering this constant frustration and conflict.

The problem is that children with AD/HD are *consistently inconsistent*. At times they can be extremely compliant and will follow your directions to the letter. At other times, however, they have a knack for pushing all the right buttons to get under your skin. The solution? Increased structure and clearer expectations will help you to become a more effective and satisfied parent.

Be honest with yourself and your family. If you're having trouble accepting the fact that your child has a disability—or you have accepted it and feel angry or guilty about it—counseling can help. You might also consider joining a support group for parents of children with AD/HD. ChADD (Children and Adults with AD/HD) has local chapters in many communities. Other support groups for AD/HD often advertise in the local activities section of your newspaper.

Many of these groups offer expert speakers as well as an opportunity to let off steam among other parents who share your predicament. What's more, studies show that over half of parents who join these groups improve their emotional well-being and feel more positive about their families and their ability to cope with AD/HD.

Above all, always try to understand your child's perspective on her problem. Just as her disability often leaves you feeling frustrated, humiliated, and guilty, she feels the same things. And, as often as you feel helpless, hopeless, and out of control, so does she. But you can't let the downside of AD/HD tear the two of you apart. Rather, you must work together to overcome the obstacles AD/HD tosses your way.

The strategies we have discussed can make a big difference at home and in the community. But they may not work all the time, particularly with children who are extremely disorganized, distractible, or active, or who have behavior problems. While moving toward improving behavior in your child, however, these strategies offer opportunities for you to alleviate some of your frustration, anger, and guilt. They are not a cure—there isn't one. But you will be amazed and pleased at how much life will improve for everyone with added structure and consistency.

CHAPTER

6

THE AD/HD CHILD
AND THE SINGLE PARENT

Debbie, a thirty-two-year-old manager for a health organization, deals with dozens of colleagues and clients every day. "But when it comes to managing my eight-year-old child, Justin, I'm at a loss," says the single mom of three.

Justin, Debbie's oldest child, has been a handful since he started crawling. Over the years, her pediatrician has suggested better discipline and counseling, and Debbie has often entertained the idea of quitting the job she loves to devote more time to the needs of her family. She has tried hard, within the confines of her harrowing schedule, to apply good discipline—and has succeeded with her two younger children. Both seem to be doing well—in fact they are prospering—with one in kindergarten and the other in second grade.

But Justin is a different story. Last year, Debbie's pediatrician suggested the possibility of Justin having

AD/HD, about which she knew little. The doctor even suggested medication, and that scared her.

Then, six months ago, life changed in a big way for Debbie. She and her husband separated, and any thoughts of leaving her job disappeared. The problems with Justin did not.

Debbie knows that Justin is a bright child, but he is barely passing most of his subjects. What's more, the constant barrage of notes from his teacher about Justin's disruptive behavior leaves Debbie feeling sad and frustrated. Homework takes her oldest son forever to complete and seems to get finished only when she stands over Justin. Meanwhile, her other children need her attention as well. And she's already pushing the limits on taking time from work to be at Justin's school to meet with teachers and administrators. Even with all this communication, nothing much has changed, and Debbie feels isolated and alone.

"I should be looking forward to coming home each day to see my children, but I get so anxious about having to deal with Justin," she admits. "When will things improve? I have fears that he will get so far out of control that I 'lose' him, plus I worry that my other children will suffer irreparably because of the amount of attention I devote to my job and to Justin. It's almost too much to deal with on my own. And their dad is no help at all—either he doesn't understand or he doesn't care."

The Two-Edged Sword: The Single Parent

When it comes to raising children, single parents face imposing challenges. Even when liberation from a failed or stressful marriage offers emotional relief, there are significant new hurdles to negotiate:

- A possible change in financial status (family income drops about 20 percent after a divorce, based on recent studies).
- Time constraints to get more accomplished in less available time—and without a partner to pitch in and help.
- Having to arrange for needed childcare and transportation.
- Dealing with the legal system for custody, settlements, and support.
- Changing residences and re-establishing social contacts.
- Finding or maintaining good employment.
- Protecting children from the stresses of divorce and from having to leave home to see the noncustodial parent.
- Facing personal isolation and feelings of loneliness.

With just one youngster to care for, a single parent often feels guilty about having enough quality time to spend with her child. With one or more additional children, stress levels are bound to soar. After all, there are so many responsibilities the custodial parent must now juggle single-handedly: getting everyone ready and off to school in the morning, preparing lunches, cleaning the house, shopping for groceries and clothes, preparing meals, getting children to and from after-school activities, making sure homework gets done, earning money, and paying bills. And when one or more of these children has AD/HD, the single parent must shift roles from dealing with just the typical stressful problems associated with parenting to the unique challenges of a parent who has a child with special needs.

The Second Edge: AD/HD

Raising normal children is an enormous challenge for a single parent. Throw AD/HD into the equation, and many—like Debbie—are at a loss what to do. She has read the material her pediatrician has given her and recognizes that delays in helping Justin may lead to more significant academic, behavioral, and emotional problems in the future. Naturally, that increases her anguish. As a single parent, how does she balance all the needs of her family while also meeting the unique and tremendous needs Justin has?

And is it really AD/HD? Debbie has seen much in the media recently about kids being overdiagnosed with this disorder and secretly wonders if maybe it's a parenting problem. Then again, she knows that Justin definitely needs more help than her other children do to get ready for school on time and to have everything packed up that he will need for the day. He often needs to call classmates after school to find out about assignments he forgot to write down or to borrow books he forgot to bring home to study. And if Debbie doesn't sit down with Justin when he does his homework, she knows that it won't be done neatly and completely.

Justin is often so wired at night that getting him to go to bed is a challenge. Once he is there, his fears often keep him from falling asleep easily. He also wets his bed periodically—which means Debbie must change his bedding regularly. With so much else on her daily to-do list, this added chore sometimes annoys Debbie. But she tries hard not to show it. She knows that her son is sensitive about wetting the bed at his age, and she doesn't want him to feel like a total failure.

So, maybe the pediatrician is right, Debbie thinks. Maybe it *is* AD/HD rather than just poor parenting. But how does she help Justin without slighting her other children—and all the while juggling the many other demands in her life?

The Right to Succeed

Both a child with AD/HD and his or her single parent have a right to live successful, happy, and fulfilling lives. However, success may very well be elusive for youngsters with this disorder who are untreated—and for their single parents, who don't clearly understand AD/HD and who fail to learn strategies to meet their own needs while also meeting the special needs of their children.

Sadly, there is no cure for AD/HD, but this disorder can be successfully managed. In addition to the many parenting strategies listed in Chapter Five, here are a few more that work especially well for single parents.

Don't Fall for These Myths

Single parents need to be aware of these misconceptions surrounding AD/HD:

Myth: *If single parents just tough it out, everything will work out okay.*

Fact: Many children of single parents experience emotional deprivation and long-term scars. Their children with AD/HD or similar problems are especially susceptible to academic and emotional problems that often follow them into adulthood. However, many behavior management approaches have been shown not only to help single parents feel more accomplished and successful with their children, but also to improve their children's performance.

Myth: *AD/HD is an excuse for poor parenting. What are needed most to alleviate the problems associated with this disorder are tougher discipline and a stay-at-home mom.*

Fact: This myth makes many parents feel guilty. Truth is, AD/HD is a medical condition whose existence has been proven scientifically. While poor caregiving and a disorganized home and family life may create symptoms that look like AD/HD, a good diagnostic evaluation, together with a knowledgeable parent and helpful professionals, can sort this out.

Myth: *Single parents are eager to put their children with AD/HD on medication just for an easy fix for their problems.*

Fact: While many parents and teachers have witnessed the benefits of medication for children with AD/HD, medication alone will not resolve the conflicts of a single parent with an AD/HD child. Nor will medication alone resolve all the problems that a child with this disorder is experiencing. Only a restructuring of how parents approach their day will help them—and their children—be more successful, happier, and more accomplished.

Establish a Routine with Consistent Rules That Can Be Negotiated as Your Child Begins to Show More Responsibility

It's tough to be the sole disciplinarian, so try involving your child in setting rules and establishing reasonable consequences for following—and not following—rules. Also consider "surveying" friends and associates or consulting other resources about ways to structure your child's morning routine, meals, homework, bedtime, and other regular daily activities. Use a trial-and-error approach to determine which strategies work best with your unique child and within your particular home setting—and stick to them.

Get Help and Support

Learn how to navigate the complex educational network of your local school system without missing excessive time from work—or feeling overstressed by school personnel whose beliefs differ from what you think your child needs. You may benefit from attending local support groups of ChADD (Children and Adults with Attention Deficit/Hyperactivity Disorders), attending community forums on AD/HD, getting books and videos from your local library or bookstore, and participating in the school PTA. By establishing friendships with supportive and knowledgeable parents who share common experiences, you, as a single parent, can avoid many errors on the way to a more successful outcome for yourself and your child.

Involve Your Child in Extracurricular Activities

Your child with AD/HD can learn to channel impulsivity and disorganization into productive activities that have a therapeutic effect both outside and inside the home. If your budget is tight, check at your child's school for free (or low-cost) extracurricular programs offered (school clubs, sports teams, and so forth). Also check local community centers for after-school programs that may interest your child. Many community programs offer transportation from school to these activities (which will save you from having to take time off from work). Some even offer free tuition or scholarships.

Schedule Quality Time with Each of Your Children

To stay on track, your child with AD/HD will require more of your attention. This is normal, and his or her siblings will probably understand, so long as they can regularly count on your undivided attention as well. How do you manage this? Try taking turns soliciting your children's help in preparing meals. Consider hiring a sitter once a month so you can take just one child out for a movie or fast-food meal. Finally, use bedtime to play "catch-up" and enjoy one-on-one conversations with each of your children.

Give Yourself Ample Duty-Free Time

Given the extra demands of supporting the success of a child with AD/HD, you need—and deserve—some time to yourself. So, do whatever it takes—sharing child-sitting duties with friends or neighbors, for example—to ensure you get at least one evening or weekend day alone on a regular basis.

The Bottom Line

Life as a single parent is a continual—and exhausting—balancing act. In addition to holding down a job, you are chief disciplinarian, housekeeper, bill payer, carpooler, nurturer, cook, seamstress, launderer—and much, much more. On top of all this, it can seem unfair to have to care for a child with AD/HD, but take heart. Armed with the right information on this disorder and behavioral approaches that work, you will gain a better understanding of how to work successfully with your special-needs child and how to negotiate home and school challenges. You will also learn to deal more efficiently with other priorities in your life.

As one parent who has risen to this challenge put it, "I'm still weary at the end of the day, but I feel like I'm doing a better job as a parent now. Not only is my child with AD/HD making great strides; I have even managed to find some time for myself. Life is definitely getting better!"

7

WORKING WITH THE SCHOOLS

Twelve-year-old Brittany has always been what her parents call "talkative and lively." So she's had her share of time-outs and missed recesses throughout her elementary-school years. "But her teachers have always tolerated her chatter, and she's always made decent grades," says Brittany's mom, Susan.

That is, until Brittany recently made the move to middle school. From day one, it's been a nightmare for her—and her parents. Oftentimes, she comes home from school close to tears and complaining that her teachers don't like her. At lunch, she claims nobody will sit with her. The papers she brings home are filled with red marks, and she's failing three subjects.

"We are very concerned," says Susan. "We never encountered these kinds of problems in elementary school. So, of course, I called to set up a conference with Brittany's teachers. And much to our surprise, one of them politely recommended that we have Brittany tested for AD/HD!"

Aside from home, school is where children spend most hours of their lives. And some children in daycare spend at least as many hours there as they do at home.

For many parents, school is simply an institution, and the only contact they have is through report cards and, perhaps, occasional PTA meetings. However, when a child has a disability, the parent-school relationship changes—often dramatically. Gone is the casual relationship that typically exists between the school and the parents of a child who is basically doing well, has infrequent behavior problems, and gets invited to parties and sleepovers by other students.

In fact, for parents of youngsters who have AD/HD, that first interaction with the school more often comes in the form of notes sent home about their child's inappropriate behavior, school work sent home to complete or redo, or a request for a conference. In some instances, this may come as a surprise to parents, whose child had not had problems before—or whose problems they had denied.

Of course, in some instances—Brittany's story is one example—it is the parents who make the first move, setting in motion a process to meet the specific needs of their child.

Regardless of who makes the first move, when your child seems unhappy at school, has red marks covering the papers she brings home for you to sign, or complains about being in trouble or having no friends, it's important to schedule an informal meeting with your child's teacher(s) as soon as possible. Even more important is that you approach this conference with one goal in mind: working with these teachers to make school as successful as possible for your child.

To make the most of this initial contact, be sure to take a list of your concerns and topics you'd like to discuss with your child's teacher. For example, maybe you'd like to address how long homework is taking, the number of "sad faces" or demerits your child has been receiving lately, incomplete classwork, missed recesses or in-school suspension, or your youngster's poor test grades—despite his seeming to know the material at home.

When setting up this meeting, be sure to allow ample time for the teaching staff to communicate their concerns as well. There should be a discussion of what factors might be contributing to your child's specific problems at school, what strategies have been used and currently are being used—both at home and at school—to address these, and what new strategies to use following the meeting.

What if AD/HD Is Suspected?

Brittany's parents admit that their daughter has always been rambunctious, but they never suspected she might have AD/HD until her teacher brought up the possibility. And, as it turns out, the teacher was right.

Keep in mind that school personnel are not authorized to make a *diagnosis* of AD/HD. They may suggest that your child's behavior is similar to that seen in children with AD/HD, but teachers should not diagnose your child or suggest a medical treatment program.

It's easy for parents to miss the signs of this disorder—especially in younger children. While often present in the elementary school years, AD/HD may not become so obvious—or cause major problems—until your child makes the transition to middle school. There, youngsters have many more responsibilities. They have to coordinate trips to their locker so they can get to each class on time. They must show up for each class with all the correct materials. They must write down homework assignments during each class, since they usually will not return to the same room that day. They also have as many as five or six different teachers—with different personalities and expectations—to please.

Another reason parents don't often suspect AD/HD is that their children, for the most part, don't cause a lot of trouble at home. Granted, they may struggle a bit at school, but parents may rationalize that maybe their child is just an average student. Or they may attribute misbehavior at school to a teacher who is too strict or to their child's "lively" personality.

As stated earlier in this book, however, an early diagnosis of AD/HD is critical to helping a child live a happy and successful life. And the good news is that, when it comes to determining whether AD/HD is the reason your child is struggling, teachers and other school personnel can help.

Teachers as a Resource

Experienced teachers are well versed in the signs and symptoms of AD/HD. But they may not always suggest such a diagnosis or recommend that a child be tested. What they are more likely to do is describe your child's typical behavior in school, then suggest you make an appointment with your child's pediatrician for an evaluation. Or they may refer you to the school's **Student Support Team (SST).**

What's that? By law, every public school is required to provide a formal mechanism to address the needs of children with academic or behavioral problems. An informal approach—that is, meetings of parents and teachers—usually is sufficient to resolve minor and temporary problems. When this approach doesn't work, however, it is often beneficial to bring together a team of individuals to help resolve the problems. Most schools call this team the Student Support Team.

An SST may be set up at the request of a teacher or a parent. To initiate this process yourself, you need only send a note to the principal requesting that a Student Support Team meeting be called to discuss the problems your child is experiencing in school.

What happens next? In preparation for the SST meeting, your child's teacher will fill out several forms that describe the problems your child is experiencing in school, list the strategies she has used to resolve these problems, and briefly discuss the success or lack of success of each strategy. Once your request is submitted, the school calls a meeting—usually within a few weeks. Naturally, you and your spouse will be invited to attend this meeting. Your child's teacher, at least one other teacher, and a school administrator will also be there. Other individuals may be invited as well, if they have information to contribute or expertise in addressing your child's needs. These may include the school psychologist, school counselor, speech and language pathologist, and special education teacher, for example.

Parents are also welcome to invite individuals to this meeting. For instance, you may want to include mental health professionals who have seen your child or a parent/child advocate who can assist you through the SST process—and in middle or high school, your child should participate on the team, as well. Formal minutes are always kept of this meeting.

What typically happens during this meeting? First, your child's problems are presented and his current performance is described. You and the teaching staff may then discuss the strategies you all have used and say which ones seem to be working, and which ones are not. If you have not already met informally with your child's teacher, expect her to bring up such issues as how rarely your child turns in all his homework and how disappointed she is that he's not studying enough for tests. You should then be ready to present your own concerns—such as how long your child is taking to complete homework, or how your child seems to know material before tests yet receives poor or inconsistent grades.

Next, expect the SST members to make recommendations based on all the information that has been presented. (A sample SST form is presented on page 118.) For example, the group may decide to try some new strategies to replace ones that don't seem to be working. They may also opt to continue strategies that appear to be helping. The team may recommend ways to boost communication between school and home. They also may suggest starting a formal testing process at school to identify factors that may be affecting or impairing your child's performance.

If you agree, this testing will be carried out at no cost to your family, but the process is often a lengthy one. For this reason, if you feel testing is necessary, you may choose to have it done privately at your own expense. It's important to remember, however, that there should be clear evidence of a learning or emotional problem before depending solely on testing, as this may delay finding the correct treatment plan for a child with AD/HD.

The SST may also recommend that you confer with your child's pediatrician or family physician for an evaluation. This will be at your expense; in fact, the school must specify that it cannot pay for these noneducational services. Finally, before the SST meeting is adjourned, a date should be set for a follow-up meeting to review your child's progress based on the recommended strategies.

Suppose the SST recommends that you have your child evaluated and you choose to have your family physician do this. When you show up for that appointment, be sure to bring along a description of your child's performance in school and a list of strategies you (and your child's teachers) have used. The minutes of your SST meeting usually contain all of this information, but you may want to supplement these with your own notes and observations. These materials should prove helpful to the physician, as we describe in the next chapter.

Once a diagnosis is made—whether your child has AD/HD or not—the SST has considerable latitude in recommendations the team can make. If the diagnosis is AD/HD, they may recommend preferential placement for your child in a class with a teacher who has particular skills or training to work with children who have this disorder. And if it's the end of a semester or school year and your child is failing some subject, the SST may

COLUMBIA COUNTY SCHOOLS   Date: ____ / ____ / _____
STUDENT SUPPORT TEAM REPORT/MODIFICATION STRATEGIES

NAME: _____ PAGE_____

____Initial SST   ____Reg. SST ____ Post Screening ____Post Psych. ____Placement

MINUTES SUMMARY

CURRENT GRADES

Rdg. _____

Spel. _____

Eng. _____

LA. ARTS _____

MATH _____

SOC. ST. _____

SCI/H. _____

CONDUCT _____

STRATEGY	REVIEW/RESULTS Date: ____ /____ /____
	Rating (1–5) C/DC Comments

agree to send your child on to the next grade despite his academic record. This usually occurs when it is clear that your child's abilities are greater than what is reflected in his report card grades.

Is My Child Eligible for Special Education Services?

Children with AD/HD may be eligible for individualized services under two federal laws: the Individuals with Disabilities Education Act (IDEA) and Section 504 of the Rehabilitation Act of 1973. To be eligible for services under IDEA, a child must have a disability that affects educational performance or learning. Many school systems deny children with AD/HD services under IDEA since they may not fit a traditional special education category, such as intellectually disabled, visually impaired, or learning disabled. In March of 1999, however, AD/HD was included in the IDEA regulations under the category Other Health Impairment (OHI). Thus, children with AD/HD who are eligible under OHI may receive modifications in testing, extra help in the regular classroom, assistance in a special education resource classroom, or other accommodations. Eligibility under OHI for a child with AD/HD usually is based on evidence that the child is exhibiting deficits in educational performance (such as poor or inconsistent grades, or impulsive or hyperactive behavior in school that interferes with learning) and verification by the child's physician of an AD/HD diagnosis.

Children who are eligible for services under IDEA will have an Individualized Education Plan (IEP) developed at a separate meeting in which you are invited to participate. The IEP is a lengthy document that specifies goals and objectives for your child's education program and what services and modifications he will and will not receive. (Samples of part of the IEP document are presented on pages 121 to 123.)

All children who are eligible for services under IDEA are

also eligible under Section 504, a civil rights law designed to prevent discrimination against individuals with disabilities. However, children may be eligible under Section 504 even if they are not eligible under IDEA. Within the school setting, the law requires that reasonable accommodations be made for children who have an identified physical or mental condition that limits a major life activity. The broad nature of Section 504 makes it an important vehicle for parents who have found the school to be unresponsive to the needs of their child with AD/HD. (A sample of a Section 504 evaluation form can be found on pages 124 to 125.)

Remember, however, that your child's success depends on cooperation between the home and school—among parents, teachers, and school administrators. Sometimes parents have unrealistic expectations for what the school should do to help their child. On the flip side, some schools are reluctant to offer individualized services for children whose success might depend on these.

Bottom line: The keys to making the relationship work to your child's benefit are good communication, knowledgeable parents, and a child-focused partnership between home and school.

Help! No One at School Is Listening!

Unfortunately, there are school personnel who are not responsive to the needs of parents and their children with AD/HD. This may emanate from lack of knowledge about the disorder, a tendency to blame parents for a child's problems, or a desire to limit the types and numbers of problems for which the school must bear educational responsibility. In such cases, we advocate the application of what we call *pleasant militancy.* This approach is intended to get the needs of your child met without alienating yourself from the school—or damaging your child's opportunities for assistance.

COLUMBIA COUNTY SCHOOLS
SPECIAL SERVICES DEPARTMENT
INDIVIDUALIZED EDUCATION PROGRAM
(IEP)

STUDENT NAME:_____ SCHOOL:_____
DATE OF BIRTH:_____ GRADE:_____
PARENT/GUARDIAN NAME:_____
ADDRESS:_____
PHONE NUMBER:_____

COMMITTEE MEMBERS PRESENT:

Name	Title	Name	Title

I. PROGRAM(S) FOR WHICH STUDENT IS ELIGIBLE:

- ☐ Autism
- ☐ Deaf/Blind
- ☐ Emotional/Behavioral Disorder
- ☐ Emotional/Behavioral Disorder - Severe
- ☐ Hearing Impairment
- ☐ Intellectual Disability -Mild
- ☐ Intellectual Disability - Moderate
- ☐ Intellectual Disability-Severe

- ☐ Intellectual Disability - Profound
- ☐ Other Health Impairment
- ☐ Orthopedic Impairment
- ☐ Significant Developmental Delay
- ☐ Specific Learning Disability
- ☐ Speech/Language Impairment
- ☐ Traumatic Brain Injury
- ☐ Visual Impairment
- ☐ Other:_____

IEP (Check as appropriate)
☐ Initial ☐ Review ☐ Addendum   Date of Annual Meeting (on or before)_____
                                                           (1 year from current IEP)

Eligibility
Current eligibility dated _____ expires _____
                        (date of most recent eligibility report)   (3 years from most recent eligibility date*)

*If eligibility expires on or before the date of the next IEP review, must address re-evaluation

☐ Eligibility re-established. Next 3 year re-evaluation due (on or before) _____
  (Complete if appropriate)   (Date)

Parent/Guardian Signature:_____ IEP Page 1 of____
Date:_____

COLUMBIA COUNTY SCHOOLS
INDIVIDUALIZED EDUCATION PROGRAM (IEP)

II. PRESENT LEVEL OF PERFORMANCE:

(Include, as appropriate, a description of the disability and its effect on educational performance; results of the most recent evaluation; strengths/weaknesses; how the disability affects the student's involvement and progress in the general curriculum; for preschool children, how the disability affects participation in appropriate activities; and concerns of the parent for the education of the child.)

Description of the disability: _____
_____
_____
_____

Results of most recent evaluation: _____
_____
_____
_____
_____

Strengths/Weaknesses: _____
_____
_____
_____

Description of how disability affects educational involvement/progress in general curriculum: _____
_____
_____
_____
_____

Parental concerns regarding education: _____
_____
_____

Additional comments: _____
_____
_____
_____
_____

Student: _____

Date: _____
Page: __2__ of_____

COLUMBIA COUNTY SCHOOLS
INDIVIDUALIZED EDUCATION PROGRAM (IEP)

VI. CLASSROOM/PROGRAM MODIFICATION RECOMMENDATIONS:

(To advance appropriately toward attaining annual goals; to be involved and progress in the general curriculum; to be educated and participate with other nondisabled students.)

A. Supplementary Aids and Services: (access to/use of)

❑ Calculator
❑ Lined paper, graph paper, lined columns
❑ Reading marker
❑ Taped materials/talking books
❑ Large print texts
❑ Note taker
❑ Other: _____

❑ Visual aids to support instruction
❑ Modified/alternative textbooks and/or workbooks
❑ Manipulative materials
❑ Times tables/charts
❑ Augmentative/alternative communication
❑ Braille texts/materials
❑ Other: _____

❑ Computer to supplement instruction
❑ Feeding equipment
❑ Preferential seating
❑ Study carrel
❑ Adaptive furniture
❑ Consult special education staff
❑ Other: _____
❑ Other: _____

B. Instructional Modifications:

❑ Secure attention before giving directions
❑ Have student repeat directions to check for understanding
❑ Material should be broken into manageable parts
❑ Avoid penalizing for spelling errors
❑ Utilize teaching assistant

❑ Directions should be simplified as needed - oral, short, specific, repeated
❑ Oral directions should be supported with written backup
❑ Check work frequently to determine level of understanding
❑ Emphasize multisensory input
❑ Avoid assignments requiring copying (writing) in timed situation

❑ Use techniques of repetition, review and summarization
❑ Provide frequent feedback and praise
❑ Remind student of class procedures
❑ Provide structured environment
❑ Modified lighting
❑ Omit contact sports/activities
❑ Other: _____
❑ Other: _____

Assignments:
❑ Written on board
❑ Extra time for completion
❑ Assignment notebook
❑ Given orally
❑ Completed orally
❑ Reduce number of spelling words

❑ Provide study guides/questions
❑ Provide extra review/drill
❑ Substitute projects for written work
❑ Reduce/shorten written assignments
❑ Reduce/shorten reading assignments
❑ Provide printed copy of board work/notes

❑ Appropriate reading level materials
❑ Provide peer assistance/peer tutor
❑ Provide individual assistance
❑ Allow difficult assignments to be completed in the resource room
❑ Other: _____

C. Student has: ❑ Special Considerations for Physical Education   ❑ Behavior Intervention Plan

VII. MODIFICATIONS FOR PARTICIPATION IN OTHER EXTRACURRICULAR AND NONACADEMIC ACTIVITIES (for which the student is otherwise eligible):

_____
_____

VIII. GRADE PROMOTION/PLACEMENT: Check appropriate statement(s).

❑ (Grades K-8) Standard promotion/placement procedures apply: ❑ Yes   ❑ No
Promotion/placement will be based on completion/progression of IEP goals and objectives: ❑ Yes   ❑ No
Other: _____

❑ (Grades 9-12) See Transition Services Plan for diploma options.   ❑ Grade placement to be determined by IEP committee.

IX. TRANSITION SERVICES:

❑ Student less than 14 years of age and transition plan not appropriate at this time.
❑ For student age 14 - 21 transition plan must include course of study. Insert page 4a.
❑ For student age 16 - 21 (or younger if appropriate) complete Transition Services Plan. Insert page 4a.

Student: _____   DOB: _____   IEP Date: _____
Teacher Signature: _____   Date: _____   Page: _4_ of ____

COLUMBIA COUNTY SCHOOLS

Section 504 Evaluation Report

Today's Date	Student's Name		
Age		Grade	Date of Birth
Parent's Name			Phone
Referral Date		School	
Reason for Meeting Today			

Evaluation Results

1. Academic Assessment Results: Evaluator _____ Date of Eval/Observ _____

2. Regular Classroom Performance: Reporting Teachers _____ Date of Eval/Observ _____

3. Social/Emotional/Behavioral Assessment Results: Evaluator _____
   Date of Eval/Observ _____

4. Medical/Physical/Sensory Assessment Results: Evaluator _____
   Date of Eval/Observ _____

5. Other Assessment Results: Type _____ Evaluator _____
   Date of Eval/Observ _____

6. Observation
   A. Observation by: _____ B. Location: _____ C. Date: _____
   D. Relevant Behavior: _____
   E. Relationship of that behavior to educational performance _____

Documentation of Eligibility

1. ☐ Student has physical or mental disability which substantially limits one or more major life activities. The disability is

_____

The disability affects the student's _____
                                                        (learning, walking, speech, etc.)

☐ Student has no physical or mental disability which substantially limits one or more major life activities.

☐ Student has physical or mental disability which does not substantially limit one or major life activities. The disability is

_____

2. Basis for making determination of disability: _____

_____

_____

3. Program Changes Needed for:

☐ Academics   ☐ Non-academics   ☐ Transportation
☐ Accessibility   ☐ Specialized Health Care   ☐ Discipline
☐ Career/Vocational Counseling ☐ Behavior   ☐ Other _____

4. Special Instructional Considerations: _____

_____

_____

_____

Documentation of Participation in This Evaluation Meeting

The following persons, as indicated by their signatures, have participated in the determination of eligibility:

Signature	Date	Position

How does this approach work? Suppose you've made every effort to get your child's teacher to help him succeed, but your pleas have fallen on deaf ears. You've tried several strategies at home that work well with your child, but when you've shared these at school, you've gotten little or no cooperation. You've made phone calls to your child's teacher, but they are not returned. You've sent notes and e-mails, but they've not been answered. Maybe you even had an SST meeting and liked the strategies they recommended, yet you don't see any evidence that these have been implemented. Meanwhile, your child continues to come home with poor grades, incomplete work, and feelings of failure. And to be honest, you share his despair!

So what's a parent to do? We recommend becoming a pleasant militant—and here's how to do that. Begin by calling the school once, twice, and even three or more times a day and asking to speak to the principal. Be persistent until you've been able to make contact. Always be pleasant with whoever answers the phone, but also make it clear that you will continue to call until you reach the principal. Eventually, the principal will respond to your calls. When that happens, it's important that your conversation not be too lengthy. Nor do you want it to be a dumping session. Rather, be ready to provide a *brief* history of the problem, state what has or hasn't been done to resolve it, and make reasonable requests for action on the school's part.

For example, you may note that your child's teacher continues to give her zeroes for homework not turned in, even though the teacher has not followed through on signing a daily homework sheet. You may relate that your child eats lunch away from the other children every day, yet the teacher has not informed you of this nor implemented a strategy to change the behavior that has led to the need to isolate your child.

You can apply pleasant militancy on the phone, in person, or in writing—whatever method makes you feel most comfortable. And, based on the response you get—and the speed at which corrective measures are taken—you can also use this approach at different levels in the school bureaucracy. All the while, be sure to keep a log of your child's successes and failures, contacts you've made with the teacher, and any other helpful information that will make communication with other school personnel more productive.

Above all, remember this: Be pleasant, be persistent, be realistic, be concise. Parents have every right to do anything possible to help their child be successful and happy. And expecting the school to share this goal is more than reasonable.

Unfortunately, in some cases of AD/HD, despite everyone's best efforts, a child's distractibility, inattention, impulsiveness, and high level of activity may persist and continue to interfere with learning and appropriate school behavior.

Then what? Keep reading, as we address complementary interventions in the next chapter.

8

MEDICATION AND OTHER TREATMENTS

Although eligible for public kindergarten, Brian was held back in preschool by his parents for an additional year. His teacher at the time suggested that Brian was immature and would benefit from an extra year in preschool. This year in kindergarten, his teacher has had frequent conferences with Brian's parents to indicate her concern about delays in his development. She says that Brian's paper-and-pencil skills are less precise than those of other children in the class, including those who are younger than he is. Neither is he learning letter names and sounds as quickly as she expects. In addition, she says Brian has trouble sitting still during story time and has more difficulty than other children staying in his learning center. When standing in line, he can't seem to keep his hands off the other children. As a result, many of his classmates have learned to keep their distance from Brian so they don't get into trouble.

Brian's parents report that at home he is always underfoot. He has trouble playing by himself and shows an interest in books and other learning materials only when someone is sitting with him. At mealtimes, he is up and down at the table and is a very picky eater. When the family goes out to a restaurant or on a shopping trip, Brian is often very difficult to manage. "He can't seem to stay in one place and often wanders off without concern for his own safety," his mother reports. His parents add that Brian is often a very sweet and sensitive child, but that they spend much of their time feeling frustrated about his inability to follow directions that seem reasonable for a child his age. They claim they have yelled, spanked, taken away privileges, and sat Brian in the corner— all with little in the way of results.

Benefits of Behavior Therapy

When a child exhibits persistent symptoms of AD/HD, the first line of defense for parents should be to initiate a behavior management program following the guidelines presented earlier. And the good news is, for youngsters with mild to moderate AD/HD, this kind of therapy can be extremely effective.

In a recent study conducted at University of Southampton in England, for example, seventy-eight three-year-olds—all boys— who had AD/HD symptoms were assigned to either a parent-training group or a parent-counseling-and-support group, or were placed on a waiting list (to serve as a comparison group). Treatment entailed a structured eight-week program involving one-hour weekly visits to a family's home made by a specially trained therapist.

Moms in the parent-training group received background information on AD/HD and were taught myriad behavior strategies to use with their children to reduce defiant and difficult behavior. These strategies included instructions on how to reward and reinforce positive behavior and ignore negative behavior. Moms in the parent-counseling-and-support group received no training, but were provided with a nonthreatening environment in which they could discuss their feelings about their child with AD/HD, as well as the impact this disorder had on their families. The group on the waiting list received no clinical services and did not participate in support group meetings.

Results? Researchers found that both groups had a significant effect on both AD/HD symptoms and the mothers' mental health. In fact, among those in parent-training groups, a full 53 percent of the youngsters improved. What's more, the positive effects of parent training were still present fifteen weeks after the training ended. In the parent-counseling-and-support group, 38 percent improved.

Most Youngsters Need More

Unfortunately behavioral interventions alone are typically not sufficient in helping the majority of children with AD/HD achieve success in their educational, social, and personal endeavors. One major problem appears to be that these strategies don't often transfer well from clinical settings to real life.

The most convincing evidence of this comes from what is called the Multimodal Treatment Study of Children with Attention Deficit/Hyperactivity Disorder. Known as the MTA Study and sponsored by the National Institute of Mental Health, this was the largest mental health study ever sponsored by the U.S. government. It followed nearly six hundred children with AD/HD ages seven to ten over a fourteen-month period.

Youngsters participating in this study were divided into four groups. Group one received stimulant medication. Group two received a combination of medication and intensive behavior therapy. Group three received behavior therapy alone. And group four received routine community care by physicians in their area using either medication or counseling.

At the end of the study, all the children involved showed

some signs of improvement—from better grades to fewer struggles with their parents. But those who improved the most were the youngsters who received a combination of individually prescribed and monitored medication and an intensive behavior management program. And the second most effective treatment? Medication alone. In fact, 68 percent of the group that received medication and intensive behavior management showed a significant decrease in symptoms of AD/HD. Compare these figures with 56 percent of the "medication alone" group, 34 percent of the "behavior management alone" group, and 25 percent of the community care group.

Does My Child Really Need Medication?

The decision to place a child on medication for what appears to be a nonmedical problem is a difficult one for parents. However, your child's current happiness and future success may well depend on your making a timely and wise decision. On the one hand, you might hope that your child will outgrow the problem quickly—or that you will learn to tolerate his difficult and stressful performance. On the other hand, your child's inability to control his behavior and to meet the reasonable expectations of school, home, and community may well lead to feelings of despair and to a resignation to being a "bad" or "dumb" child.

Many studies show that the longer-term outcome for a child who has adopted this low self-image can be dismal. While parents may choose to assume the role of martyrs by putting up with their youngster's difficult behavior, it does a child little good in the short term—or the long term. For this reason, you shouldn't be surprised if your physician prescribes medication designed to modify the neurochemical errors in your child's brain. And take heart! As many as 80 percent or more of children with AD/HD who take medication show improvement—and without harmful side-effects.

Types of Medication for Children with AD/HD

When your child's doctor recommends medication, what is he most likely to prescribe? Actually, there is no one-size-fits-all prescription for AD/HD. In fact, many different kinds of medications have been used successfully with children who have this disorder.

To determine which one may be best for your child, a physician will use a symptom profile of your child along with clinical experience. That means your input about your child's home performance—and input her teacher provides about school performance—can be extremely helpful in allowing the doctor to make an informed decision.

Regardless of what is prescribed, the goal—as with almost any medicines—should always be to use the lowest possible dosage that produces improved behavior. And if an initial regimen doesn't seem to be working, don't be alarmed if your child's physician recommends changing the dose, adding another drug, or switching to another medication to see what works best.

Stimulant Medications

Oddly enough, stimulant medication appears to be the most effective therapeutic approach for treatment of AD/HD—especially when combined with behavior management strategies. Why does stimulant medication work on a child who may already appear overstimulated? While it may seem counterproductive, stimulant medication is believed to work by blocking the reabsorption of certain neurotransmitters, notably dopamine, from the synapse before nerve impulses can cross from one nerve cell to another in particular parts of the brain. When the neurotransmitter remains in the synapse, the nerve impulse can cross the gap more efficiently. In fact, the changes induced by stimulant medication manifest themselves in decreased impulsiveness and hyperactivity and improvement in a child's attention span. Children with AD/HD who take stimulant medication also are less aggressive and more compliant, and enjoy improved motor skills.

Methylphenidate Hydrochloride

Methylphenidate hydrochloride has been the most frequently used stimulant for children with AD/HD. It has a long history of use and a high success rate, and it results in relatively few and minor side-effects.

Until recently, Ritalin was the most common brand of methylphenidate hydrochloride prescribed; now several new forms have been introduced. Ritalin is supplied in a short-acting and a longer-acting sustained released (SR) form. Ritalin LA is the newest Ritalin formulation on the market and offers the rapid onset and a long-acting effect. A typical starting dose is five milligrams (5 mg) once or twice a day of the fast-acting medication with adjustments, and additions later in the day for after-school use. Pills are available in 5-mg, 10-mg, and 20-mg doses. Ritalin takes effect within about thirty to forty-five minutes and usually lasts for three to four hours. These pills may be cut in half to adjust doses on the recommendation of your physician.

The 20-mg SR form cannot be cut or divided and often requires a little longer to take effect, but it should last approximately seven hours. The absorption of the SR dose often is less consistent than that of the fast-acting dose. Benefits from using an SR dose may include fewer behavioral peaks and valleys during the day and elimination of a noontime dose—of particular value to middle- and high-school students who are sensitive to the stigma of taking pills at school. A single-dose approach, which was first introduced with this SR dose, is also of value when the child does not get the pill at school consistently. Often, fast-acting Ritalin is added to an SR dose to provide the best coverage through the day.

For many decades, Ritalin was the only brand name that delivered methylphenidate. Recently, however, several other forms of the same drug were introduced, which use different delivery systems. Concerta comes in a three-chambered capsule. The outer coating of the capsule is fast-acting methylphenidate that is activated soon after the capsule is ingested. One of the chambers of the capsule contains a polymer substance that expands as it absorbs fluids from the digestive tract. As it expands, it gradually pushes out methylphenidate contained in the other two chambers. Concerta is supposed to last ten to twelve hours, but actual response duration varies in different children. The capsule comes in doses of 18 mg, 27 mg, 36 mg, and 54 mg, with a 72-mg dose planned for release in the near future.

More recently, Metadate ER was introduced. It is similar to Ritalin SR, and comes in 10-mg and 20-mg doses. It lasts about eight to nine hours. Metadate CD is a newer delivery system for methylphenidate. It comes in capsule form and contains beads of methylphenidate. Depending on the coating of the bead, the drug is released at different times following ingestion of the capsule. Approximately 30 percent of the medication is released immediately. The remainder is released gradually over the next ten to twelve hours, according to the manufacturer. Once again, actual response duration will vary from child to child. Metadate CD comes in doses of 20-mg capsules.

Finally, Focalin is a short-acting refined form of Ritalin that isolates the effective isomer of methylphenidate. It comes in doses of 2.5 mg, 5 mg, and 10 mg and is intended to be given in divided doses of 5 to 20 mg per day. It is formulated so as to reduce the side-effects common to stimulants. And since it uses only the more active of the isomers, lower doses may be effective.

A new Methypatch should be available soon. The small patch would be worn on the skin under one's clothes. Since it will not go through the digestive system, lower doses should be possible. Also, the drug dose should drop immediately when the patch is removed. This might be beneficial for students with irregular schedules and for workers with irregular work and sleep schedules.

Amphetamines

Dextroamphetamine (Dexedrine and Dextrostat) was once a very popular drug for use with children with AD/HD. Once available in elixir form, which made it a desirable option for very young children, it was the only medication approved for preschool-aged children. With other safe medications available now, dextroamphetamine is used much less often now than in the past. Dexedrine and Dextrostat come in fast-acting forms in doses of 5-mg and 10-mg tablets. Dexedrine also comes in a longer-acting spansule, which releases half of the dose in about one hour and the other half about three hours later. Response duration is approximately six to eight hours and varies from one individual to another.

Dextroamphetamine is one of four amphetamine salts contained in a relatively new and frequently used medication, Adderall. The mixture of salts, each of which acts over varying lengths of time, provides duration of action of as long as eight hours. In one recent study, teaching staff were asked to monitor youngsters with AD/HD who were taking stimulant medications. Response of the children to Adderall was significantly more positive than response to Ritalin, in a ratio of three to one. Adderall tablets come in various doses up to 30 mg and are double-scored for easy adjustment of dose based on your physician's recommendations.

Recently, a newer form of Adderall was introduced. Adderall XR comes in capsule form in doses of 10 mg, 15 mg, 20 mg, 25 mg, and 30 mg. The duration of action is as long as twelve hours. Half of the dose is administered rapidly and the other half approximately four hours later.

Side-effects for all these stimulants are the same: headaches, abdominal pain, lethargy (tiredness), tachycardia (rapid heart rate), difficulty falling asleep, loss of appetite, tics, and mood swings. Some of these side-effects diminish as a child adjusts to the medication, but you should always share serious concerns with your child's physician, who may change the dosage or switch to another drug.

The movement clearly is toward single-dosing of children in the morning to carry them at least through the school day and, in many cases, through after-school daycare, homework, and recreational activities. Single-dosing clearly is beneficial in that it eliminates the need for taking medication at school. Not only is there the stigma of others' knowing that the child takes medication, but according to a recent survey of more than five hundred parents of children with AD/HD, almost 100 percent feared that their youngsters wouldn't receive the right dose of medicine at school. The good news is that, with the availability of many different types of medication and durations, doses can be tailored to the specific needs of your child's and family's schedule.

One major reason stimulants are considered so safe is that they act quickly and are not stored in the body. Maintaining therapeutic blood levels over time is not required. That means children who can do well in nonschool activities may not need to take medication on weekends.

An exception to all of this is Cylert (pemoline). Cylert was touted as one of the first longer-lasting medications for children with AD/HD. It comes in tablets in doses of 18.75 mg, 37.5 mg, and 75 mg with duration of action of approximately eight to ten hours. It also comes in a chewable form. Side-effects include those normally found with stimulants. However, recent evidence has shown a risk of serious liver damage. Therefore, Cylert is used infrequently and only when other proven treatments have not been effective.

Stimulants: The Great Debate

In that survey involving over five hundred parents of children with AD/HD, nearly nine in ten said their child had been given a prescription for stimulant medication. But only half of those youngsters were taking it.

What gives? Unfortunately, many newspapers, magazines, and television talk shows have attempted to sensationalize stimulant therapy. Naturally, this alarmist approach has triggered an impassioned debate, and parents aren't sure what to believe.

Are stimulants prescribed too readily? That's tough to say. Some three million American schoolchildren have taken Ritalin and other stimulants, and the number of prescriptions for these drugs has jumped about 400 percent since the early 1990s. Studies also show that children in the United States are ten times more likely to receive a prescription for stimulants than are youngsters in Europe—and twice as likely as children in Canada. Yet, as University of Massachusetts Medical Center psychologist Russell Barkley, Ph.D., points out, "The U.S. leads the world in psychiatric research, so we have simply moved ahead of other countries."

Claims of rampant overmedication may be unsupported as well. According to a recent study involving almost thirteen hundred children with AD/HD and their parents, only about one in eight had been given stimulant medication.

A majority of physicians who have prescribed stimulants, as well as parents of children who have used these medications, will tell you stories about how they have changed youngsters' lives for the better. "We noticed a dramatic change in the very first week," says one mother of a child with AD/HD. "For the first time in years, our son could sit still at the dinner table, pay attention in class, focus on his homework, and carry on a real conversation with me. It was an amazing transformation!"

Decades of studies on stimulant medications support this anecdotal evidence. In other words, there is conclusive scientific evidence—over sixty years' worth—that a vast majority of youngsters with AD/HD enjoy clearer thinking and calmer behavior after starting these medications.

Nevertheless, myths and misconceptions persist and, before you agree that your child with AD/HD try stimulant medications, you should know the facts. (See the box below, "Setting the Record Straight.")

Monitoring Your Child on Stimulants

Any physician will tell you that stimulant therapy works best when parents take charge and closely monitor their child's progress. Here are some guidelines we recommend following as your child begins his treatment plan:

Let Your Child Know Why He Is Taking Medication

Children from the first grade on are aware that they are experiencing difficulty concentrating, controlling their behavior, being organized, getting along with other children, and so forth, and they are often consoled to know that medication may resolve these problems.

Setting the Record Straight

What are some of the misconceptions surrounding stimulant medications?

Myth: *Stimulants cause dangerous side-effects ranging from permanent brain damage and severe depression to growth retardation and Tourette's syndrome.*

Fact: There is no scientific evidence to indicate that stimulant medications cause brain damage or severe depression. But, as with all medications, individual children respond in different ways to the same type and dose of medication.

The most common side-effects of stimulants are decreased appetite and insomnia. Other side-effects include headaches and stomachaches. In rare cases, a child may experience extreme agitation or rapid heart rate. Side-effects often cease after the body adjusts to the medication or with a decrease in dose or change in medication.

Tourette's syndrome may be unmasked as a side-effect of stimulant medication. The medication does not cause this disorder; in fact, since Tourette's syndrome is a hereditary condition that involves vocal and motor tics, there is usually a family history of the disease. Notify your child's doctor if the disorder exists in your family, so that he can closely monitor your child's use of stimulant medication or prescribe an alternative medication.

Myth: *Stimulants aggravate hyperactivity in children with AD/HD.*

Fact: Occasionally, a parent may notice what experts call a rebound effect in their child when the medication is wearing off. The youngster appears extremely restless and may be more difficult than ever to control. This usually occurs in the late afternoon and can last for thirty to forty-five minutes. It doesn't mean that your child is reverting to a premedication state. Nevertheless, many physicians who once limited their AD/HD patients' dosages of stimulants to school hours are now prescribing an extra dose late in the day to help youngsters maintain control through the late afternoon and early evening or using extended-release medications that will last through more of the day.

Myth: *Stimulants cause children to exhibit "zombielike" behavior.*

Fact: Stimulants, by nature, do not have a tranquilizing effect. However, too large a dosage may cause a child to be lethargic. Consequently, if your child appears glassy-eyed or complains of feeling overly tired and down in the dumps, his dosage likely needs to be adjusted. Be sure to contact your physician should this behavior persist.

Myth: *Stimulants are addicting.*

Fact: There is no evidence to suggest that this is true for children with AD/HD when they are carefully monitored. In most instances, youngsters remain on the same dosage for years; in fact, some may get by with a lower dosage as they grow older. Furthermore, when children with AD/HD forget to take their medication—or their parents opt not to administer it on weekends or vacations—children show no symptoms of dependence.

Myth: *Taking stimulants puts children at greater risk of becoming drug or alcohol abusers later in life.*

Fact: Because children with AD/HD are more impulsive, they may be more prone to experiment with drugs and alcohol. But it's their disorder that puts them at risk, not their medication. In fact, studies at Harvard Medical School found "absolutely no evidence" that youngsters treated with stimulants became teenage substance abusers. Results were similar in another study involving more than two hundred boys at New York University's Child Study Center—and this one followed youngsters well into their thirties.

What's more, some studies suggest that the opposite is true. That is, children with this disorder who receive stimulants are less impulsive and thus, less likely to experiment with drugs and alcohol. Proof: Researchers at the State University of New York at Stony Brook followed two groups of children with AD/HD from the 1970s to the mid-1990s. One group was treated with stimulants; the other was not. By the end of the study, researchers found that the youngsters who took stimulant medication had *lower* rates of substance abuse as they grew up! In other words, when stimulants have a positive effect on a child's behavior, he feels more in control of his life and receives more positive feedback from others. As a result, his self-esteem soars, which makes substance abuse far less likely.

Occasionally, your physician may suggest that neither your child nor his teacher be told why your child is taking the medication. The reason for this "secrecy" is to help prevent what is called a "treatment effect." This occurs when a person knows that he is being treated for a certain condition and that the treatment is expected to cause certain changes. Sometimes the person expecting a change will alter his behavior voluntarily or subconsciously and cause some changes to occur, regardless of the actual effect that the treatment has or doesn't have. To avoid this treatment effect, physicians may ask that the participants in a medication trial be kept "blind" to the expected changes that the medication should have. Once this trial period is over, however, your child and his teacher can be made aware of the reason for the medication.

It is important that a child understand that the purpose of the medication is only to help her do her best. The medication should never be used as "the reason" for good performance or behavior. Neither parents nor teachers should suggest that the child's medicine "must have worn off" or that "It must be time for your medicine" when behavior becomes more difficult. Children must learn to be responsible for their own behavior rather than to depend on "outside forces" to control them. So, treat the medication as a part of your child's daily routine without drawing unnecessary attention to it.

Keep in Mind that There Is No Clear Rule Regarding How Much Medication Is Needed by a Given Child to Achieve Desired Results

Children of the same size or age may require significantly different doses to achieve the same benefits. Moreover, as time goes on and as children grow, it is quite common for them to "outgrow" a dose and for a regression in behavior to occur. If and when this happens, an adjustment in the dose may be necessary.

Sometimes, even after a brief positive response to the medication, regression may occur, requiring your physician to adjust the dose. On the other hand, many children learn to compensate as they get older and mature. Increases in dose may not be needed and, in fact, some children may succeed on a lower dose or no medication. But only a physician should adjust the medication dose.

Also, keep in mind that medications are typically started at a low dose and increased gradually until an effective dose is achieved with the fewest side-effects. With some medications, the correct dose may be achieved in a matter of days; with others, it may take several weeks.

Recognize that Dose Is Often Related to School Demands

Parents may find that their child on medication does well before the winter school holidays and then shows regression in performance when school begins again in January. Their thinking is that the medicine isn't working anymore. In fact, what may be happening is that the work demands have changed. Many elementary schools, for example, use the first few months of the school year to review material from the previous year;

then the pace and intensity of work increase beginning in January. Faced with such an increase in academic and organizational demands, a child who had been doing well before the break with medication and behavior management may no longer have a medication dose sufficient to meet these increased demands.

Similar problems occur when a child moves from elementary school to middle school. In the former setting, she had one or two teachers and usually stayed in one classroom. In the latter setting, she may have more than half a dozen teachers and move from class to class with stops at the locker during the day. Again, whereas a certain medication dose and behavior management strategy were sufficient in elementary school, an adjustment might be needed to meet the more intensive demands.

Work with Your Child's Teachers to Monitor Your Child Closely for Side-Effects and Report Any Concerns to Your Physician

Side-effects are not usually serious with these medications—especially at the dosages used for children with AD/HD. Nevertheless, they do occur. The most common side-effects are headaches, stomachaches, lethargy (tiredness), tachycardia (rapid heart rate), persistent difficulty falling asleep, persistent loss of appetite, tics, and mood swings. Some of these side-effects diminish as the child adjusts to the medication. But you should always share serious concerns with your child's physician.

Follow the Prescription Directions Carefully

None of the typical medications taken for AD/HD comes in chewable form. In addition, medications should not be cut, split, or ground up without your physician's express orders, since this might affect the potency and consistency of action of the medication. If you have questions about the medication or how to get your child to swallow a pill, talk with your physician or pharmacist.

Avoid Attributing Normal Developmental Behavior Patterns to the Medication

Once a child starts medication, parents often become alarmed by every behavioral episode that breaks the normal routine. Parents should realize that most children get into occasional fights, sometimes have sleepless nights, may not like what is served at mealtime or are not hungry, fail to bring home a book, or even blow a test. Only when a *pattern* of old behavior appears is it time to consider what might be causing it and talk to the teacher, your physician, or a psychologist or counselor to figure out how to get your child back on track.

Always Give the First Dose of Stimulant Medication on a Weekend

That way, you can monitor any immediate side-effects and look for positive changes. If your child takes medication only for school, you get little feedback from the teacher, or the medication wears off by the time he gets home, you may think the medication is not working. Therefore, it's best to start the medication when you have a chance to see how it affects behavior, how long it lasts, and whether it affects your child's appetite or sleep patterns or causes any other side-effects.

Always Follow your Physician's Directions Regarding How Much Medication to Give to Your Child and When to Give It

Be sure to provide feedback on the ups and downs of the child's day, at different times of day, in different settings, and in different activities. Don't ever adjust the dose on your own.

After a trial period, tell your child's teachers that he is taking medication so that they can be on the lookout for side-effects and report improved performance. Maintain close communication with the teachers. Resist attempts to attribute every poor grade or breach of rules to the medication. Children with AD/HD are children first and aren't perfect!

Some children do fine on one dose of medication per day; others need additional doses to stay focused throughout the afternoon and evening. Keep your physician informed with concise and precise information about how your child responds both to the medication and to behavior management strategies in different activities and at different times of day.

Medication for Nonschool Activities

Should your child take medication on weekends, holidays, after school, and during the summer? The traditional thinking was that the medication need only be used during school hours. That thinking has changed dramatically. Typically, physicians now make this decision based on how well your child functions in his environment without the medication, balanced against the significance of side-effects. For example, if your child exhibits poor self-control at restaurants, family outings, or at church or synagogue, continuing her medication might be advisable. Similarly, if your child spends her time during soccer and softball games watching birds fly overhead or digging holes in the ground with her foot, it might be advisable to try her on medication during these times.

Again, though, this decision must be balanced against the undesirable side-effects that increased medication may have. If taking it late in the day interferes with your child's ability to fall asleep at night, or it causes such a dramatic decrease in appetite that there is a significant weight loss, your physician might choose to withhold medication, alter the dose, or consider other medication options.

Medication often is critical during homework and study time. A few brief assignments may take several hours to complete, and studying may be a wasted effort for a child who is too distracted and fidgety to focus on the material. This also is a time of day when everyone in the home is tired and has a shorter temper. Together with behavioral interventions described elsewhere in this book, homework and study times are appropriate for a medication trial to see what benefits are realized. In other words, if homework time is typically spent arguing with your child, medication at this hour can enhance family harmony. It may also provide your child with the extra time needed for recreational activities, time that he might otherwise spend anguishing over getting his homework done.

When trying to decide whether your child needs medication during homework and study time, consider these questions and share your answers with your physician:

- Is my child working efficiently? Is she learning the material and can she remember what she has studied?
- Is homework and study time notable for constant conflicts and stress?
- How effective are behavioral approaches in getting homework completed correctly and in a reasonable amount of time?

As we indicated earlier, by "reasonable" we mean no more than two to two and one-half times the amount of time that primary-grade children are expected to spend on homework and no more than 50 percent more than the amount of time middle- and high-school students are expected to spend on homework. If your child consistently requires at least that long or longer to complete his work—and requires your constant attention to help him finish it—it is appropriate to talk with your physician about the use of medication.

In sum, children who have a considerable amount of homework and studying each day, are involved in many afternoon and weekend social and athletic activities, or create conflicts at home or in groups may benefit from being on medication throughout the day and week. The ability to perform well in a given setting is a critical factor in a child's short-term and long-term success, as is the supportiveness of his family. Medication can play an important role in enhancing a child's performance and making home life more peaceful.

Other Medications

SNRI

Atomoxetine, marketed under the brand name Strattera, is the first nonstimulant medication specifically for the treatment of AD/HD. Atomoxetine is a selective norepinephrine reuptake inhibitor (SNRI) that was originally used as an anxiety and depression medication. Since it is not a stimulant, prescriptions are not limited to one month at a time. In addition, results of a few studies performed with atomoxetine indicate success with children and adolescents, and provide evidence of benefits in social, family, and school performance. Side-effects are similar to those experienced with stimulants.

Many other medications are used for children with AD/HD, often to address coexisting conditions. Some of these are described below.

Antidepressants

Certain antidepressants have been prescribed as sole medications for some children with AD/HD. For example, the tricyclic antidepressant Tofranil (imipramine), when administered at low doses, has been found effective in some children at controlling symptoms of AD/HD and bedwetting. At higher doses, it controls depression, although it is not used as a first-line medication for depression in most cases. Imipramine is provided in doses of 10 mg, 25 mg, 50 mg, and 100 mg and should provide twenty-four-hour coverage, based on the individual.

Wellbutrin (buproprion) is another antidepressant that can have a positive impact on AD/HD. Like imipramine, buproprion affects the neurotransmitters norepinephrine and dopamine in much the same way that stimulants do.

Selective serotonin reuptake inhibitors (SSRIs), including Prozac, Paxil, and Zoloft, often are used in combination with stimulants for children who have AD/HD and depression. While by themselves they have little impact on AD/HD, the mode of action of SSRIs on the neurotransmitter serotonin is similar to that of stimulants on other neurotransmitters.

With all antidepressants, the medication must be taken daily and the child must be weaned off the medication when the physician recommends discontinuation.

Antihypertensive Medications

Two medications, approved for a very different purpose, have been found useful for addressing certain aspects of AD/HD and coexisting conditions. Catapres (clonodine) and Tenex (guanfacine) may improve hyperactive, impulsive, and aggressive behavior. They also appear helpful for improving symptoms of oppositional defiant disorder (ODD). For children who have difficulty falling asleep as a side-effect of stimulant therapy, these medications improve symptoms of insomnia. Catapres and Tenex also appear to reduce facial and vocal tics in Tourette's syndrome. When discontinuing these medications, the child must be weaned off gradually to avoid sudden changes in blood pressure. Catapres is available in pill and patch form. Tenex is available only in pill form.

Antianxiety Medications

Relaxation techniques and cognitive behavior therapy may provide some help for older children with anxiety that coexists with AD/HD. There are unique medication problems when these conditions exist together. Children with AD/HD and anxiety show a decreased response to stimulant therapy compared to children with AD/HD alone. These children appear to do better on certain tricyclic antidepressants (such as Tofranil, Norpramin, or Pamelor), benzodiazepines (such as Ativan, Klonopin, or Xanax), and BuSpar.

Mood Stabilizers

For children who have bipolar disorder and AD/HD, mood usually must be stabilized before symptoms of AD/HD can be addressed. Mood stabilizers such as Tegretol and Depakote have been effective with children with this disorder. Then, once the effectiveness of mood stabilizers has been determined, stimulants are usually added.

All of these medications for treating coexisting conditions have potentially more significant side-effects than stimulant medications. Therefore, it is important to closely follow your physician's directions for safe use and to report any unusual responses you observe or that your child relates to you.

Medication for Life?

Youngsters who take medication to help control AD/HD continue this therapy for different lengths of time. Deciding if and when medication should be stopped is based on your child's ability to control his behavior on his own. In other words, as he matures and becomes more aware of his behavior, he may find himself more in control.

In general, by the time a child with AD/HD reaches kindergarten or first grade, he is aware of his behavior, but he is not yet equipped with the skills necessary to maintain control of himself. By fourth grade, children's self-awareness is far more heightened, and peer pressure becomes a factor as well. Consequently, at this age, youngsters may begin to show levels of self-control and self-discipline to compensate for AD/HD during nonmedicated times. This is very dependent upon the environment in which the child was raised and neurological issues, however. If self-esteem has remained high and the child's errors have been forgiven and redirected, he is more likely to learn from those errors and apply energy toward self-control. Of course, the only way to determine whether a child can get along without medication is to compare his performance in similar situations on and off medication. For this reason, physicians often plan intermittent drug holidays to observe how the child handles himself in various settings without medication.

By helping to keep children focused and in control, medication can have a tremendous impact on children with AD/HD. But their treatment cannot stop there. In fact, sometimes the rapid improvement in a child's attention span has unpleasant outcomes. He may become more aware of his academic problems and more attuned to the difficulties he has experienced with other children. This can lead to increased sadness and even signs of depression. Or, he may begin to show a keen interest in new activities his parents consider insignificant.

Neither of these situations should alarm parents. They simply demonstrate that, to reach their fullest potential, children with AD/HD need time as well as support and supervision from both their parents and others outside the home, such as school counselors, educational administrators, teachers, and coaches.

Remembering Medication at School

The issue of remembering—or being willing—to take medication is an important one for children who are scheduled to take medication at school. Some schools prefer placing responsibility on the child to remember to go to the office to get his medicine. However, it is because of the child's poor organizational skills and his forgetfulness, in part, that he is taking the medicine! Therefore, placing the responsibility on the child is setting him up for failure.

Making teachers responsible for a child's taking medication has its drawbacks as well. They often have so much going on in the classroom at once that they may forget to remind the child that it is time for his medication. Teachers also may have many children in the class who take different medicines on different schedules. Keeping track of each child becomes a difficult process.

Several approaches can be used to help ensure that your child receives his medication daily:

- Tie taking medication to a specific daily activity. For example, have your child stop at the office for his medicine on the way to lunch, on the way back from the computer lab, and so forth.
- Ask the school nurse (if there is one) to help remind the child and monitor the regular dispensing of the medication to him.
- Consider buying your child a digital watch with an alarm. Set the alarm for the time when the child is to report to the office for his medication. Be sure that his teacher is aware that the watch will beep at that time and that the purpose is to make the child responsible for following his own schedule.

Adolescents taking these medications present another problem. One of the characteristics of this age group is a sense of invulnerability. For example, they may decide that they no longer need or want to take medicine. They may also be reluctant to attribute failing grades and increased behavioral problems to their decision to quit taking their medicine. In such instances, parents should try one of these approaches:

- **Reasoning:** Call your child's attention to the increased problems he's been having since stopping the medication. Or, on a trial basis, agree to let your child not take the

medication but compare his performance on and off medication for no more than half a grading period (from
report card to progress report or vice-versa).

- **Contingencies:** Tie privileges to taking the medication.
  For example, your child gets to use the computer, borrow
  the car, or go to the movies with friends only if you see her
  take her medication that morning.

- **Routine:** The most desirable approach is to maintain taking medication as a "nonevent" in the child's life. That way,
  no attention is called to it, and it becomes a part of the
  daily morning routine without much ado.

- **Consultation:** Set up a time for your child to talk with
  your physician, school counselor, religious leader, or psychologist. A professional may have specific skills and expertise that will convince your teen of the need to take his
  medication regularly.

Controversial Treatments

Several kinds of treatments that are considered controversial are
currently being used for children with AD/HD. Many of these
approaches have been scrutinized by researchers and scientists
and found to be lacking in a number of ways. And while often
supported by anecdotal information from parents, their success
has not been documented in published research reports.

Documentation published in research journals satisfies a
number of requirements that should be met before acceptance
of a treatment. First, it provides a specific description of strategies used in treatments. This information helps practitioners
gain a better understanding of the conditions under which a
certain approach may or may not work. Second, it describes
the individuals on whom the strategy was used. The success of
the strategy with a certain segment of the population does not
necessarily mean it will be useful with other individuals. Third,

published research should compare the results of using an approach to changes in the individual when the approach is not used. This practice of using "controls" allows practitioners and other scientists to look at the actual changes that occur when the approach is used and to compare them with variations and changes that occur naturally over time or to other scientifically accepted strategies.

Fourth, to conclude that an approach works, a large and well-defined sample must be used and appropriate statistical analysis applied. Fifth, research papers are traditionally submitted to other professionals for their review and critique before a paper is published in a journal. This peer-review process provides a standard whereby research reports that do not meet the necessary professional criteria generally will not be published and consequently will avoid misleading readers. Finally, documentation should also contain evidence that other individuals who use the same approach have achieved the same results. If one researcher reports that a certain technique works but no other researcher is able to duplicate the results, it provides false hopes for parents and skepticism among professionals.

Often, controversial treatments are presented in books that appeal to the lay public only. The author of the book usually is the developer of the treatment approach, which, in itself, should give parents pause. After all, the developer of a truly worthy treatment would be eager to have the effectiveness of the treatment proven by sound research. Tales from a few satisfied users hardly represent the millions of individuals who might benefit from a valuable treatment.

Many different approaches fall into the category of controversial treatments:

Neurofeedback

Advocates of this approach indicate that the child can be trained to alter brain electrical activity. Specifically, proponents believe that attention, focus, and concentration can be improved, together with task completion and organizational skills, impulsiveness, and mild hyperactivity, through an intensive training program whereby the child's brain activity is shown on a screen similar to an electroencephalogram. The child is then taught to alter the brain waves in a way that would enhance attention and would decrease symptoms of AD/HD. The few published reports available on this treatment, however, do not clearly define how the treatment is used. Nor do they use large enough sample sizes or control groups. Replication of results has also been insufficient to support the widespread use of this expensive approach.

Diet

Diet therapy to treat AD/HD has received greater attention from the media than have treatments supported by published research reports. Unfortunately, there is little evidence—aside from anecdotal reports—that an additive-free diet, a gluten-free diet, an allergen-free diet, an antioxidant-rich diet, or any other idea that calls for removing or adding certain food items (such as sugar) or using supplements (such as pine bark extract or shark oil) makes any consistent difference in the child's behavior. In fact, sound research studies that have examined the effects of diet on characteristics of AD/HD consistently do not support the broad success of a dietary approach for children with AD/HD. This does not necessarily mean that you shouldn't consider trying a dietary approach. There probably are a small percentage of children who, in fact, would benefit from diet modification. However, diet management should fall under the supervision of a physician who will monitor the child's general health, weigh the child regularly, and might conduct periodic blood tests. In any case, the wise parent is one who naturally limits the quantity of "empty foods" that a child eats anyway.

Orthomolecular Approach

Advocates of this approach believe that certain genetic abnormalities produce alterations in the child's need for, or metabolism of, certain vitamins and minerals. Unfortunately, there is little consistent support for the strategy of providing children with AD/HD with vitamin and mineral supplements. No well-controlled studies support the approach. Both the American Psychiatric Association and the American Academy of Pediatrics have stated that supplements make no difference in the behavior of a child with AD/HD.

Yeast Control

Another proposal is based on the idea that at least some of the behavior associated with AD/HD is due to excessive growth of yeast in the body. The excessive growth of yeast results from a weakened immune system or from treatment with antibiotics, which kill bacteria that normally keep yeast growth in check. Supporters believe that this excess of yeast produces toxins that hinder the immune system and cause AD/HD, among other problems. Consequently, proponents of this approach recommend the use of medications—such as Nystatin—to control yeast growth. However, no research to date supports this claim.

Sensorimotor Integration Therapy

Two recent approaches relate to the vestibular system, which is made up of the organs of the inner ear and the cerebellum. Advocates of these approaches believe that problems with this system cause poor integration of brain functions and consequent organizational problems and other difficulties. One approach recommends the use of anti-motion sickness medication or antihistamines combined with stimulant medication. The other is based on sensory integration theory. In brief, this theory proposes that nerve pathways in the cerebrum, the thought-processing and information-storage part of the brain, can be altered by stimulating the vestibular mechanism in the ear. While this particular approach may work with some children who have certain kinds of learning disabilities or neuromuscular problems, there is no scientific evidence that either of these approaches benefits children with AD/HD.

DHA Supplements

There is some research suggesting that brain levels of docosahexaenoic acid, or DHA, are low in children with AD/HD. Since DHA tends to concentrate in the membranes of nerve cells, especially where they contact each other, this theory sounds plausible. However, in one recent study, more than sixty youngsters with AD/HD randomly received either DHA or a placebo for four months. Results? No differences were found in the two groups, according to subsequent psychological tests and rating scales completed by parents of these children.

Acupuncture and Chiropractics

These approaches are based on the belief that putting pressure on points along the energy pathways of the body or adjusting the alignment of the spinal column can curb impulsiveness. But, again, there is no scientific evidence to support these notions.

Cognitive Interventions

A number of cognitive strategies have been proposed that claim to decrease a child's impulsiveness and improve attention and self-control. The most successful of these is self-monitoring, in which children are trained to track and monitor their own behavior. Other approaches—such as self-instruction and anger-control training—appear to be ineffective. In fact, most cognitive strategies tend to transfer poorly from clinical to real-life settings. By themselves, they tend to yield unsatisfactory outcomes. They may be of use, however, when combined with other treatment approaches.

Parents Beware!

Many individuals have grown wealthy preying on the frustrations of desperate parents. There are always people hopeful that the next "solution" that comes along will be the answer to their problems. Please be cautious and conservative when someone claims to have a cure for AD/HD. The truth is that there are no cures yet for the disorder, and that is not likely to change for quite some time.

Nevertheless, for children who don't respond to traditional scientifically proven approaches, using other strategies that will not harm the child and may work is reasonable. Relaxation therapies—such as meditation and yoga—for example, have been shown to help some children with AD/HD, particularly those who suffer from anxiety. And such classes as tae-kwon-do, a form of karate, can be helpful since they teach children to focus their attention and follow instructions. Just don't disregard safe approaches in favor of alternatives that are unproven. After all, the future of your child is at stake!

CHAPTER

9

THE ROLE OF TEACHERS

Jenny, a fifth-grader, has missed recess for nearly two consecutive weeks. Her teacher knows how much Jenny likes to play outside and is trying to encourage her to earn back this privilege. The problem? Jenny's name has been on the board every day for nearly a month— for not turning in her homework assignments on time, for turning in incomplete classwork, for talking too much in class, and for picking on the other children in her class at lunchtime.

Jenny's teacher is confused. She sees Jenny win class spelling bees and can't understand why she consistently scores in the low 70s on written spelling tests. She watches Jenny complete math problems perfectly on the board and is confounded when the majority of Jenny's answers on written math tests are incomplete or incorrect. She is always telling Jenny, "I know you can do better," yet Jenny insists that she is trying as hard as she can.

158

Just like the parents of children with AD/HD, teachers also experience confusion and frustration about these children's attitudes and abilities. And with good reason. In some instances, the child with AD/HD appears bright, capable, and motivated; in others, she appears lazy and uncommitted to accomplishing her goals and objectives. Because of this inconsistency, some teachers instinctively blame the child for her poor and sloppy work, repeatedly insisting, "I know you can do better than that." Or they point the finger at the child's parents and encourage them to be more firm and strict with their offspring.

Parents, in turn, will tell their youngster's teachers how hard they have worked to support their child with AD/HD. They will explain how they have attempted to be more restrictive by depriving their children of privileges, by putting them in time-out and, in some cases, by spanking them. None of these measures, they will likely add, has worked effectively. They will also recount the number of hours they have spent helping their child finish a homework assignment that should have taken just minutes to complete.

The problem is that, unless teachers fully understand what AD/HD is and how it affects its young victims and their families, they cannot appreciate that the child's problem is with what she *shows* rather than what she *knows*. For example, once teachers realize that the child can work well on an individual basis and orally, they will learn to credit the child when she demonstrates her skills in these ways. Teachers with a solid knowledge of AD/HD and its effects will also soon discover that results of traditional testing typically understate what the AD/HD child has learned. Most important, once a teacher finds the flexibility and strategies to help the child with AD/HD succeed and feel successful both academically and socially, the child and her parents will feel encouraged as well.

Parents as Educators

Children with AD/HD are constantly on the receiving end of messages from adults that say, "You are a problem and a disappointment." Consequently, when teachers write messages on the paper of a child with AD/HD such as, "Sloppy—do over," when it was the child's best efforts, or, "This is easy work—you need to study more," when the child and her parents spent hours the night before preparing for the test, it reinforces the child's feelings of incompetence and leaves the parents feeling exasperated. As a result of these persistent messages over several years of schooling, the child eventually becomes resigned to the fact that she is incapable of meeting her own—or anyone else's—expectations.

Many of these children eventually give up their unsuccessful attempts to please others and to accomplish personal goals. Some may become oppositional and then exhibit severe conduct problems. Others may begin to show signs of apathy, anxiety, and depression. Still others look for reasons to avoid work, such as repeatedly getting up to go to the bathroom, sharpen their pencil, or get a drink of water. Moreover, some children, whose impulsive behavior leads them to do things that are contrary to their value systems (such as stealing), may begin lying as a defense mechanism to preserve some degree of self-esteem.

That's why it is critical for parents to make sure that their children's teachers not only understand AD/HD but also do all they can to help those children succeed in their classrooms. Most teachers are familiar with AD/HD but many do not know the cause or its effects or how to implement strategies that can improve these children's behavior and performance. That's where you, as a parent, can help.

First, make sure that your child's teacher has a thorough understanding of AD/HD. A good first step is sharing "What is

Attention Deficit/Hyperactivity Disorder? A Guide for Teachers" (see page 162) with each of your youngster's caregivers and instructors at the beginning of the school year. Next, establish a good working relationship with your child's caregivers and teachers. Let them know that you are able and willing to serve as a resource for them by providing suggestions for strategies they can try in the classroom to help both your child and others with AD/HD succeed. Make it clear that you will monitor your child's progress very closely. Engage in *pleasant militancy* if supportive approaches are rebuffed. Finally, study the "Strategies for Success in the Classroom" section in this chapter carefully so that you can serve as a knowledgeable advocate for your child—and as a resource for his teachers.

Keep in mind that your child's response to the different approaches a teacher uses to solve problems in the classroom will vary based both on the severity of your child's problem and his age. Therefore, you may find that one or two of the strategies we discuss will help to resolve many of the classroom problems your child is experiencing. Or you may discover that using all of the strategies still does not bring your child up to a level of performance high enough that he experiences academic success or increased feelings of self-worth. Nevertheless, it is the teacher's obligation to try classroom modifications before suggesting a Student Support Team meeting or a consultation with a physician. And while you don't want to be pushy when suggesting some of these ideas to your child's teachers, you may have to be politely firm and insistent.

Also keep in mind that middle and high school make the advocacy process for your child more difficult. You may wish to sit down very early in the school year or just before the start of school with all of your child's teachers to discuss the modifications that will be most helpful. If necessary, the school counselor or assistant principal usually can facilitate setting up such a meeting.

What Is Attention Deficit/Hyperactivity Disorder? A Guide for Teachers

Attention Deficit/Hyperactivity Disorder (AD/HD) affects between 3 and 5 percent of all school-age children. More boys than girls have higher ratings for inattention, impulsiveness, hyperactivity, and externalizing problems, such as conduct disorders. Girls with AD/HD have greater intellectual impairment and internalizing problems, such as depression.

There are three types of AD/HD. One is characterized by hyperactivity and impulsiveness. These youngsters are generally easy to identify in the classroom. They are out of their seats frequently, move around the classroom more than other children, and have trouble staying in one place. They tend to be bossy and have trouble getting along with their peers. Children who have AD/HD characterized by chronic inattentiveness, on the other hand, may be more difficult to pinpoint. The most common characteristics to watch for include daydreaming, not completing seatwork, difficulty getting started on seatwork, poor organizational skills, and frequently losing and forgetting things.

Children with a combined type of AD/HD show characteristics of both inattentiveness and hyperactivity/impulsivity.

Children with AD/HD have difficulty following instructions; forget to write down homework assignments, even after being reminded repeatedly; don't hand in assignments, even when they have been completed; and don't appear to be motivated, as other children are, by incentives. Dig a bit deeper, however, and you may be surprised to find that the child is capable of doing more than a superficial evaluation indicates. For example, if you call on a child with AD/HD when she appears to be daydreaming, she often has the right answer. If you sit down with her to redo a unit test on which she received a 42, she may surprise you by getting a 96. And if you call her up to the chalkboard to do a problem that she missed on a worksheet, she is likely to answer it correctly. These discrepancies in performance make it imperative for teachers to be particularly patient and understanding with children who exhibit symptoms of AD/HD.

Very often AD/HD occurs in conjunction with other problems. For example, many children show impairment in written language (penmanship, spelling, grammar, and fluency), spoken language (including word retrieval and fluency), memory, and reading. Some children meet the diagnostic criteria for depression, oppositional defiant disorder, anxiety, and other disorders. Some disorders are genetically linked to AD/HD; others are a by-product of the inattention and poor motor control one finds in children with AD/HD. Relationships with some problems are still unknown. The good news is that the symptoms of some of these secondary problems sometimes improve when AD/HD is successfully treated.

Help Is Available

In recent years, school systems have made many resources available to you, in both print and other media, to help you work with these children in your classroom. In addition, the Student Support Team structure helps to provide better communication within the school system by assisting with monitoring the child's progress, by preparing him or her for formal psychoeducational testing, if needed, and by offering a way to get the child's parents involved in more structured ways to deal with the comprehensive needs of the child.

What to Look For

What can you do if you suspect that a child has AD/HD? Find out all you can about working with a child with AD/HD so you can implement useful strategies in your classroom. Eventually, you may suggest that the parents talk with their physician based on what you have observed about the child and his response to the strategies you have used. When should you suspect AD/HD? There are a number of checklists available that assist in testing your suspicions. Keep in mind, though, that *AD/HD is a medical diagnosis that can be made only by a physician.* Most physicians, however, will welcome and solicit your input in helping to differentiate between AD/HD and other problems that may manifest similar types of symptoms.

An AD/HD Checklist

The following questions can assist you in validating your suspicions that a student has AD/HD. All evaluations are made relative to other children of the same age.

1. Does the child appear to daydream or is he easily distracted?
2. Does the child have difficulty sustaining attention on tasks, particularly seatwork?
3. Does the child have difficulty getting started on seatwork?
4. Does the child often fail to complete work but give responses at the beginning of the task that are often correct?
5. Does the child consistently respond better orally in class discussions than on paper-and-pencil evaluations of the same material?

6. Does the child fidget a lot, playing with papers, pencils, zippers, and so forth? Does she assume unusual postures (legs folded under, half-standing and half-sitting, and so forth)?

7. Does the child perform better one-on-one and in smaller groups than he does when working independently or in a whole-class activity?

8. Is the child impulsive, doing and saying things before he thinks? (This may include calling out in class, pushing another child, providing off-the-topic answers to questions, and so forth.)

9. Does the child have difficulty getting homework assignments written down, taking home the correct books for homework and studying, carrying notes back and forth between home and school, and so forth?

10. Has the child not responded consistently to being held in from recess, to assertive discipline strategies, and to incentives for improved performance?

11. Does the child do poorly on class work and often not hand in homework even though his parents indicate that they spend considerable amounts of time working with the child each evening at home?

There are many variations in the performance patterns of children with AD/HD. For example, many children do extremely well on tests even though their day-to-day performance is extremely poor. However, if the answer to most of these questions is "yes," it is advisable to assume that the child has AD/HD and to implement appropriate strategies until a definitive medical diagnosis is made.

Strategies for Success in the Classroom

Getting Teachers on Your Side

When parents suggest that individualized strategies be used in working with their child with AD/HD, teachers are often concerned that other children will feel left out or slighted. Fortunately, this is an empty argument. Children are often far more insightful than adults and are quick to realize individual differences in their peers. In fact, they often become one another's strongest allies. Therefore, when help is provided to a child who has difficulty staying in her seat, finishing her work, or participating in classroom activities without undue disruption to the class, her classmates will understand. For most children the satisfaction of completing a task, getting a good grade, and "fitting in" is sufficient reward to keep them happy and productive in the classroom. When additional intervention is needed for one or two other children in the classroom, they will raise no objection.

In applying intervention strategies, suggest that your child's teachers start with one strategy and try it for several days before evaluating its success. After that, another strategy can either replace the first or be added in stepwise fashion until your child's performance improves to an acceptable level compared with other children in the class—or until all strategies have been tried and been found to be unsuccessful. Obviously, you'll have to rely on the teacher's judgment to determine the best combination of strategies, how long to continue with each one, and how to make them work for your child in her classroom. So, be sure to touch base with the teacher periodically to see how things are progressing.

For children in upper elementary grades and beyond, where several teachers are involved, make sure that all of your child's teachers use similar strategies for the same types of problems—unless, of course, your child's problem is manifested in different ways with different teachers. In that case, each teacher should use strategies that best meet the individual needs of that classroom, teacher, and your child. In middle school and high school, it is often wise to identify one contact person—a homeroom teacher, school counselor, or assistant principal—with whom to maintain contact.

Preferential Seating and Proximity Control

Placement in the classroom of a child with AD/HD should be chosen carefully. Some children will perform better when seated near the teacher or paraprofessional's desk. Others will do best sitting closest to the chalkboard or in the front of the room. Still others will perform better when they are seated in the middle of the classroom or near other children who can serve as work models for them. Most will do best away from windows or doors where visual and auditory distractions abound. In any case, the teacher may have to try several seat locations before finding one that works best. And placement may have to change many times during the school year. The criteria for successful placement should be: improvement in copying materials from a chalkboard, beginning work more quickly, staying on task to complete seatwork, paying attention during teacher-led activities, and decreased distractibility and inappropriate interactions with other students.

Proximity control also is beneficial in maintaining a child's attention on task and controlling nonproductive behavior. These strategies include standing near a child, looking at her, and touching her shoulder. Using a child's name during a lesson also is very effective for keeping a child's attention—asking, for example, "How long would Holly take to travel 420 miles if she was in a car going sixty miles an hour?" Hearing her name, Holly is tuned back in to the lesson.

Rehearsal

The wise teacher uses preventive strategies to ward off potential problems with children whose behavior tends to be difficult. For example, the teacher may take a child aside as he comes into the room in the morning to remind him of the morning routine. As the child leaves the room to go to the bathroom, the teacher may remind him about bathroom rules. As the child is lining up to go to physical education or recess, the teacher should ask him what the rules are at these activities. "I want to be proud of you and I want you to be proud of yourself for following those rules," she might say to the child. Working with children to rehearse correct ways of behaving in different settings helps them to be more successful by avoiding problems.

Increased Vigilance During Unstructured Times

Social problems (pushing, throwing objects, taking objects from others, and so forth) among children who are impulsive tend to increase during the less structured times of the school day—transitions from one activity to another, during lunch, between classes, while at recess, and in physical education class. Therefore, during these times, greater supervision by adults can often head off potential problems and prevent a child with AD/HD from making a foolish mistake. The child should be at the teacher's hip walking down the hall and the recess supervisor should gaze in the child's direction every few seconds to be sure the child is playing nicely. Quick intervention can prevent a problem from occurring. The child should be reinforced for playing well during recess, for walking down the hall calmly, and so forth. Don't let good behavior go unnoticed.

Study Buddy

With twenty-five or more students in a class, teachers often have a difficult time giving a distracted child the amount of attention needed to keep her working productively. Furthermore, when a child's name is repeatedly called out and accompanied by negative messages, it can be equally frustrating to both the child and the teacher. Often, making statements such as, "I like the way _____ is working" (using the name of another child who is demonstrating good work habits), will help the child with AD/HD get back on task. But even this may be a futile effort in the long term. Therefore, seating the child next to an ambitious but subtle student is often beneficial. Give responsibility to that child to assist the youngster with AD/HD to stay on task, have the correct materials out, and keep the right place during class activities. The ideal study buddy is one who can do this in a matter-of-fact way without calling undue attention to the student.

Organizing Work

There are a number of ways a teacher can assist the poorly organized child in getting started on seatwork or in completing assignments. First, worksheets or assignments can be numbered, so that, rather than shuffling papers or books for twenty minutes in an effort to decide which to do first, the child completes them in numerical order. Second, the child can be given just one worksheet or assignment to complete at a time. When it is completed, she delivers it to the teacher or paraprofessional, who gives approval to move on to the next task. Third, the child can keep a list of assignments on her desk, then check these off as she completes them. Although a similar list may be on the chalkboard, the nearness of an individualized list may be necessary to help the child with AD/HD become better organized.

Finally, a timer may be placed on the child's desk and set for a reasonable amount of time for her to finish a given task. In one classroom, the teacher had a box full of timers that were available to any child who wanted to use one. This destigmatized the use of the timer by the child with AD/HD by making the modification socially acceptable. Often the visual reminder provided by the timer, along with a specific allotment of time provided, will help a youngster with AD/HD get started on a task more quickly and complete it more efficiently. The amount of time to provide for a task should be left to the discretion of the teacher. However, it should be long enough to assure the child an opportunity for success but short enough to provide a mild challenge. As days pass and the child achieves success, the amount of time should be shortened for similar types of tasks.

Adjusted Workload

Many children with AD/HD are easily overwhelmed both by papers with a great deal of writing on them and by complex tasks. While the intent of reducing a child's workload is not to have lower academic expectations of her, it may be necessary—at least initially—to reduce the amount of work the child must do to demonstrate that she knows the concepts that are being taught. On math worksheets that have twenty-five problems to complete, for example, the last ten problems may be no more difficult than the first fifteen. Therefore, if the child completes only ten to fifteen of the problems rather than all twenty-five, she is still demonstrating knowledge of the math concepts.

Similarly, if the class must write or correct ten sentences to indicate a mastery of appropriate punctuation, the child with AD/HD can demonstrate the skill by doing half of those sentences. The purpose of this approach is to allow youngsters to experience success, while acknowledging that they have mastered the skill or concept but are unable to sustain attention long enough to complete the longer assignment. Over time, of course, the intent is to increase the workload as children show increasing ability to do longer assignments. In addition, youngsters should learn to self-monitor their quality of work and task completion during this process.

Grading Work

It is frustrating for a child to try his best and continue to earn poor grades because he is unable to complete work. When a child with AD/HD shows a consistent pattern of incomplete papers and assignments, encourage the teacher to either cut down the length of the work or grade only what your child has completed. This provides your youngster with an opportunity to get graded for his knowledge and skill of the material rather than for his inability to sustain attention to his work. An alternative to this approach is to have the teacher hand the paper back to your child at a different time and allow him to complete the rest of the assignment without penalizing him. It is important to recognize that, for preschool children as well as high-school children, it is disheartening to consistently receive sad faces or red F's marked on papers when the child is making his very best effort and really knows the material but is unable to control inattention and distractibility.

Unfinished Classwork

If your child is not completing work in the classroom and thirty minutes of homework is already taking two hours or more to complete at home, a teacher sending home additional work to complete merely transfers the crisis from the classroom to the home. This also places an unfair burden on you and unrealistic demands on your child, who should have some time each day for recreation. Parents often look to teachers as the experts in dealing with these kinds of problems. But when the teacher shifts that responsibility back to the parents, it breeds greater frustration and anger in parents, who may feel "dumped on." In such instances, you'll need to work closely with your child's teacher to negotiate ways in which your youngster can complete enough of his work to be graded fairly, but not so much that he is forced to become a young—and frustrated—workaholic.

Incentive Systems

Teachers of young children often use incentives such as stickers, end-of-week parties, and other treats to motivate students to do their best. For children with AD/HD, the rewards for doing work may need to be provided on a shorter-term basis, and the menu of incentives may need to be varied. For older children, the types of incentives may need to be modified (special computer time, the chance to act as bus monitor or raise and lower the school flag, and so forth), but the use of incentives can still be effective for increasing productivity and feelings of self-worth.

There are many approaches to incentive systems. All variations focus on the child's positive behavior and efforts rather than on breaches of the rules alone. Offering desirable incentives with reasonable expectations for performance lets children feel that they can be successful and even benefit from extraordinary efforts.

▪ **Immediate tangible rewards.** A child may receive a tangible reward, such as a sticker, for completing a specific task or assignment within a given amount of time or for demonstrating a particular behavior such as staying seated for a specific amount of time. The criteria for success should be challenging yet reachable. For example, a child may get a sticker each time he stays in his seat for at least a fifteen-minute period or for each worksheet he completes during seatwork time. As a parent, you can assist by providing the teacher with ideas for incentives to which your child is likely to respond.

▪ **Token economy systems.** A token economy system offers immediate feedback with delayed gratification. In this system, children receive a token or marker to indicate that they have met some criterion. However, youngsters must accumulate a certain number of markers before receiving a reward. These markers may be lines drawn on an index card on a child's desk, Popsicle sticks, buttons, and so forth. The child then has a menu of rewards for which he can cash in these markers when he has accumulated enough of them. The menu should have items with different point values and should consist of tangible items and activities that the child particularly enjoys. These might include stickers, pencils, time at the computer, a trip to the library, an opportunity to read to kindergarten children or to be a peer tutor, a trip to the principal's office for a treat, or a free homework pass. The token economy system for positive behavior is a valuable one to try, particularly when the name-on-the-board approach and missing recess do not work. Menu items should be varied weekly and created in consultation with children so that items that are most valued by the youngster are on the menu.

Classroom Segregation

At times, separating a child with AD/HD from the rest of the class may decrease distractions and provide the youngster with greater control over his work habits. It is best for teachers to deal with the issue in a straightforward way. In other words, they should talk with the child about his tendency to have trouble getting work finished when he is with the group and offer him the opportunity to sit at a table or study carrel positioned in a way so that there are fewer visual and auditory distractions. When reading groups are going on, for example, the child should be placed as far away from the reading group as possible to complete seatwork. Otherwise, the auditory distraction will hinder productivity. Similarly, a special table can be turned to face a corner or wall so that the number of visual distractions is limited. In general, the child should have the opportunity and freedom to go to that table when he feels it is necessary to complete his work. Some youngsters, however, may need to be encouraged to move to the table when it is apparent that they are not completing their work.

For many children, the use of a study carrel with barriers in the front and on the sides—or a cut-out refrigerator box with the desk placed in it—may be useful. To destigmatize its use, the teacher should give other children an opportunity to use it for specific projects and tasks. Allowing a child with AD/HD an option to work while standing or using a lectern or high table may improve productivity as well. After all, the purpose of segregation in the classroom is not to punish the child but to allow him opportunities to be more successful and to teach him how to modify his own environment to enhance productivity. The child is free to return to the group when he feels he's ready to work productively with his classmates.

Cooperative Groups

Children with AD/HD often benefit from opportunities to work productively with their peers in small groups. Clear rules for group work should be established, since youngsters with AD/HD appear to do better with increased structure. Group work allows for positive peer interaction, and smaller groups help enhance a child's attention to the learning tasks.

Homework

When it comes to homework, many problems plague children with AD/HD. They often forget to write down homework assignments. They forget to bring home the books they need to complete their homework, and they often take three to four times as long as other children to finish the same homework assignment. Moreover, when they complete their homework they often forget to pack it in their backpack or to hand it in the next day. Here are some strategies you and your child's teacher can try:

▪ **Homework pad.** Most children have a special place where they write down their homework assignments. In the early grades, teachers often provide a photocopied sheet that indicates the assignments for the day or for the week. For the child who consistently leaves school without his assignment written down, the teacher will probably need to see that the child has a sheet like this and that it goes into his backpack. Or the teacher needs to look at the written assignment entered on the child's homework pad and initial that it is complete and correct. Expecting that a child will remind his teacher to do this at the end of the day is setting the child up for failure. Think about it. The child is using this strategy because he forgets to write down the assignment. So it is just as likely that he will forget to ask the teacher to sign the pad. Therefore, at least initially, the teacher or paraprofessional should be encouraged to remember to ask the child for the pad—or a peer should be assigned to check the child's homework pad.

- **Missing materials.** Children who rarely remember to bring home the right books for homework or for studying, or children whose desks consistently overflow with papers that should have gone home days or weeks earlier, should be instructed to empty the contents of their desks or lockers into their backpacks daily. While this may be a physical burden, it ensures that all books and papers a child needs to take home leave the school. As youngsters become more successful at demonstrating responsibility in the classroom, they can be weaned from this task.

- **Location of homework assignments.** If your child is doing his homework at night but the teacher claims that he is not handing in assignments consistently, call a strategy session with the teacher. Work together to devise a system whereby your child's homework papers will be placed in the exact same place in his backpack every night when he is finished with his homework. That way, if the child doesn't hand in the homework on his own, the teacher or your child's study buddy can check in that specific location every morning to find it.

- **Limited homework time.** As noted earlier, children with AD/HD can take hours to complete a brief homework assignment. Yet parents feel obligated to ensure that the child does all his homework and feel guilty when he goes to school with unfinished assignments. Find out from your child's teacher how long homework should take. If you are consistently spending more than twice that much time to help your child finish his homework, suggest that modifications be made. The most reasonable approach is to see that your child spends no more than two to two-and-a-half times as long on homework as other elementary schoolchildren and not more than 50 percent longer than older children. You might send a note to the teacher indicating how much time was spent on the homework and that it was not completed in that time frame. Your youngster can then be graded on what he completed or be given an opportunity to complete the homework in class.

Teachers can also help you find appropriate ways to structure your home environment so there are incentives for the child to get his homework done as quickly and correctly as possible. For example, maybe your child should not be allowed to go outside to play, watch television, play video games, or drive the car until his homework is done. However, when your child is unable to complete his homework in the allotted time—even with these incentives—modification should be made in length of assignments.

Specific Instructional Strategies

Tannock and Martinussen, writing in *Educational Leadership,* conceptualize AD/HD as a learning rather than a behavioral disorder. They describe specific teacher strategies to promote academic success.

- **Teacher talk.** The teacher uses strategies such as modeling, repeating, elaborating, and defining. Since children with AD/HD frequently have difficulty understanding directions and expressing themselves, the teacher rephrases the student's language so as to provide a model for future use and to make statements more understandable and useful to peers. Furthermore, linking difficult concepts to concrete images often helps the student to remember material more easily and efficiently.

- **Teaching social skills.** Children with AD/HD often have poor social skills. Reduction of negative responses from their peers through enhancement of skills such as turn taking can increase cooperative learning opportunities for them.

- **Changing the level of support.** Lessons may need to begin in a teacher-directed format where material to be learned is modeled. Gradually, through a period of guided practice, the child takes more control of the learning process.

- **Providing instructional supports.** Teachers can influence the learning environment in their choice of individual versus group instruction, the use of cues, the types of correctional strategies that are applied, and the use of visual aids and mnemonics. These approaches reduce the demands on working memory, which may be faulty in a child with AD/HD.

Daily Report Card

It's unrealistic for teachers to expect parents to control their child's behavior or work habits in the classroom. After all, parents are not usually there to see what goes on. Logically, a school's professionals should address events that occur during the school day. There may be times, however, when linking school and home performance is necessary. A good example is when school incentives do not appear to be working, but the child has many activities to which she looks forward at home each day. On these rare occasions, using a Daily Report Card may prove useful. The Daily Report Card is a type of token economy system that offers home consequences for school performance. (Examples of Daily Report Cards for

DAILY REPORT CARD — Elementary School

Name:_____   Week of: _____

★★

	CLASSWORK	BEHAVIOR	HOMEWORK*	COMMENTS	
MONDAY	2		Letter review worksheet. Complete and return.	Parent's signature:	**MONDAY**
TUESDAY	3		Letter review worksheet. Complete and return.	Parent's signature:	**TUESDAY**
WEDNESDAY	4		Numeral writing. Complete and return.	Report Cards in folder. Return the envelope. Keep the report. Parent's signature:	**WEDNESDAY**
THURSDAY	5		Practice writing your name (first and last).	Parent's signature:	**THURSDAY**
FRIDAY	6		No homework.		**FRIDAY**

*Stamp if yesterday's homework is handed in.

DAILY REPORT CARD FOR MIDDLE-SCHOOL AND HIGH-SCHOOL STUDENTS

Name: _____   Date: _____

CLASS	CONDUCT (Circle)	CLASSWORK (Circle)	HANDED IN HOMEWORK?	TEST GRADES	COMMENTS	T. INITIALS
Period 1	S U	S U	Y N			
Period 2	S U	S U	Y N			
Period 3	S U	S U	Y N			
Period 4	S U	S U	Y N			
Period 5	S U	S U	Y N			
Period 6	S U	S U	Y N			
Period 7	S U	S U	Y N			

elementary-, middle-, and high-school-aged children are presented on pages 178 and 179.)

In general, here's how a Daily Report Card works. The teacher rates the child at the end of each class or school day on the basis of class work performance, conduct, and whether or not the child handed in homework completed the previous night. Grades of A, B, C, D, and F, S (Satisfactory) and U (Unsatisfactory), or a stamp are given. If a child receives all satisfactory grades, she earns all privileges at home that day once her homework is completed. This may include going outside to play, watching television or playing video games, or borrowing the car to run errands. If the child gets one unsatisfactory grade for that day, however, she loses the most valued privilege at home for the remainder of that day. Finally, if the youngster receives more than one unsatisfactory grade or comment, she loses all privileges and must go to bed early that evening. The next day, the child starts over with a clean slate.

What do you do if your child fails to bring home the form, claims the teacher did not fill it out, or offers any other excuse for why she could not present it to you? Treat this as if there were unsatisfactory grades or comments on the form. This teaches your child responsibility and prevents the use of excuses to avoid consequences.

Student Support Team

School systems in every state are obligated by law to have a Student Support Team (SST) structure. Teachers who have been actively involved in the SST process know that the success of the team depends on the leadership of the group and on the openness of members to carefully analyze each child's problem and consider all possible alternatives. For the child with AD/HD who has no indications of a mental handicap or learning disability, interventions may include those described in this chapter or, in rare instances when a teacher cannot or will not implement reasonable strategies, a change of class.

As described earlier, the SST is also the pipeline for psycho-educational testing and special education services. Granted, children with AD/HD often do not qualify for traditional types of special education classes. But a case of AD/HD that does not respond to intervention and that seriously impairs the child's ability to learn may make a child eligible for special education services under the Other Health Impairment category or for services under Section 504 of the Rehabilitation Act. In any case, the SST process should focus on involving all parties productively in helping the child to be more successful in school-related activities.

Managing the Child on Medication: The Teacher's Role

Teachers play a vital role in managing children who take medication for any reason. When a child is prescribed medication for AD/HD and it is not taken as directed or is omitted altogether, it is not the physical health of the child that suffers but her self-esteem, as well as the tone of the whole educational environment. The teacher's personal feelings about medication should be put aside when she is faced with a child who is not responding to behavioral intervention and who clearly is not meeting expectations.

As discussed in Chapter Eight, many types of medication are used with children who have AD/HD. While many come in a time-release form and some can be administered by a transdermal patch that the child wears, some of these drugs must be administered several times a day.

Physicians will often begin children on medication by way of a blind study. That is, they may start the child on medication without the teacher knowing it, or they may intersperse the real medication with a placebo to determine the true effect of the medication. It is extremely important, therefore, that your child's teacher watch carefully for alteration in your child's behavior within a given day, as well as from one day to the next. A logbook or log sheets often serve as excellent documentation to verify the difficult behavior the child exhibits, as well as to later reflect any benefits that the child shows from various types or doses of medication. This log should also include comments about the child's activity level, her ability to pay attention and work, and interactions with her peers. The teacher should begin a log as soon as she notices unusual behavior and prepares to begin an intervention strategy. (An example of a teacher's logbook appears on page 183.)

Many children who are anxious about school complain about headaches, stomachaches, and other problems. Children with AD/HD often are among this group. Therefore, it may be difficult for teachers to differentiate the complaint of a child experiencing side-effects from AD/HD medication from those of children who see school as a frustrating and unpleasant place. The most common side-effects of medication used for AD/HD are headaches and stomachaches, loss of appetite, lethargy, and increased irritability. Communicating this information to your child's teachers and educating them on what to watch for will enable you to compare their input with information provided by your child's physician regarding side-effects for the type of medication your child is using.

When children are supposed to take medication several times a day and forget to take a dose, both your child and those around her may suffer. Missing a noontime dose of Ritalin, for example, may cause increased distractibility and activity level during the afternoon hours, as well as generally poor performance. It is important that your child take medication at the prescribed times, even though it may interfere with her participation in a classroom activity or be difficult for a teacher to remember to send her to the office to get her medicine. One way to help a teacher out in this regard is to suggest that your child take her medicine routinely in conjunction with a change in activities. Maybe she could stop by the office on the way to lunch every day or on the way back from the computer lab. You may also get your child a digital watch with an alarm, which can be set for the time when she should go to the office to get her medicine. Work with your child's teachers to devise strategies that draw as little attention as possible to your child when she must take her medicine and find ways to place as much responsibility as possible on your child to monitor herself in taking it. Keep in mind, though (and remind the teacher), that the reason your child is taking the medicine is for the very problems that may prevent her from remembering when it's time to take it. Expecting your child to remember on her own consistently is setting her up for failure.

Sample: Teacher's Logbook

2/6 (Wednesday)

Amy was ten minutes late to school. Seemed in good spirits but did not turn in all of her homework. Sat quietly and listened well when guest speaker spoke to class. Seemed alert and asked the speaker good questions. During lunch Amy was reprimanded twice—once for breaking in line and once for talking too loudly at the table. After lunch Amy appeared restless and could not seem to concentrate on her math test. Handed in her paper with only half of the test completed. At recess Amy and a classmate were put in time-out for calling each other names. After recess Amy performed well in class spelling bee but couldn't settle down after that. She kept getting up to sharpen her pencil, get water, and so forth.

2/7 (Thursday)

Amy on time this morning but turned in only half of her homework. Seemed very tired. Said she didn't sleep well last night. Fell asleep at her desk during morning seatwork. Barely touched her food at lunch. Said she wasn't hungry. After lunch complained of headache. School nurse gave her some Tylenol. Amy seemed irritable the rest of the day. Asked to sit out during PE. Didn't seem interested in any classroom activities today.

2/8 (Friday)

Absent.

2/11 (Monday)

Good day overall. Turned in her homework. Sat quietly and watched movie with rest of the class in the morning. Enjoyed music class. Helped me put up a new bulletin board before lunch and seemed pleased with her contributions to the effort. Ate well at lunch. Played well with peers at recess. After lunch was a bit restless during social studies. Finished nearly all of her math problems. Volunteered to play the lead in a class play we're planning. Became hard to manage as we were preparing to go home. Had to be told several times to pack her backpack and straighten her desk.

2/12 (Tuesday)

Another good day. Turned in all of her homework. Was proud to make the highest grade in the class on a spelling test. Behaved very well on our class field trip. Had minor problems at recess when classmates made fun of the way she played kickball. Worked hard for nearly an hour writing an essay for social studies. Did not finish her essay but asked if she could complete it at home overnight. Behaved extremely well in art class.

A Final Word

Children with AD/HD cannot succeed in school without the understanding and flexibility of their teachers. Moreover, children's experiences in school affect both their life at home and their future. Therefore, it is your role as parents to do all you can to ensure that teachers are educated about this disorder and are sensitive to the impact their approaches have on these special students.

AD/HD is not just the child's problem. It is not just the parents' problem. Nor is it just the school's problem. It is as pervasive and as potentially debilitating as the most severe mental or physical disability. It takes away a child's desire to face a challenge, strips him of his self-esteem and self-respect, and may even cause him to question his reason for living.

As teachers become more informed about the disorder, they will be better able to help children with AD/HD experience success in spite of it. They will be better able to help youngsters with AD/HD understand, accept, and compensate for their shortcomings. And they will be better able to offer you sensitivity and hope.

CHAPTER

10

THE CHILD GROWS UP: LEAVING HOME

Caroline, seventeen, is a junior in high school with dreams of going to college and eventually becoming a teacher. Diagnosed with AD/HD in the fifth grade, she struggles to keep her grades up. She scored well on her SATs, thanks to the extended time she was given to take the test. Now she's begun the process of filling out applications to several colleges.

Her number one choice is a large state university about one hundred miles away from home. But Caroline's mother worries about her daughter's chances of succeeding in classes with 150-plus students. She also thinks a huge campus—with so many activities going on—may be too distracting.

What's more, Caroline has recently been skipping her stimulant medication, insisting she can get along just fine without it. Meanwhile, her mom has serious reservations that Caroline will be able to cope in college without it.

Most children leave home around the age of eighteen. Some head off to college or technical school; others join the military or find jobs. And this rite of passage is almost always a source of pride for parents, who have devoted many years to preparing their children for adulthood.

But the moving-out process can also be bittersweet for everyone involved. There is excitement, for sure, but it's not unusual for both parents and children to feel anxious and apprehensive as well.

This is especially true of parents of a child with AD/HD, who can't help but wonder and worry, "Will my child be able to succeed in the real world?" The good news is that if these children have received appropriate treatment for their disorder, parents have every reason to be optimistic.

Preparing Your Child for College or Technical School

These days, postsecondary education is a ticket to higher wages. But before you begin searching for colleges or technical schools for your child with AD/HD, make sure that's what he wants to do. Youngsters with AD/HD must often work extra hard and spend more time on course work than other students—and if your child isn't motivated to do this, you may be wasting his time and your money.

If your child is committed to higher education, however, here are some strategies that can help ensure his success.

Know Your Rights

Section 504 of the Rehabilitation Act of 1973 says that institutions receiving federal funds (almost all colleges and technical schools do) must provide reasonable accommodations and academic adjustments to any disabled students. To take advantage of this law, however, you must provide the school with documentation of your child's disorder (for example, a note from your child's physician or psychologist). Your child will then be eligible for special assistance. Some schools, for example, will provide note takers, tape recorders, special test-taking provisions, tutoring, and even increased communication between the school and you.

Look for a School that Will Be Supportive of Your Child

Despite the law, not all schools will provide the services your child may need to succeed. So, when checking out schools, always contact the office of the dean of students and arrange a meeting with whoever is in charge of services for students with disabilities. That way you can ask specifically what modification programs are available for students with AD/HD.

Keep in mind, too, that as a rule of thumb, youngsters with AD/HD fare better at smaller schools—at least initially. Fewer students in classrooms usually means instructors are more approachable, have an opportunity to get to know their students better, and provide more personalized attention. Smaller campuses can also be less overwhelming and provide fewer distractions.

Of course, once your child adjusts to college life, she can always transfer to a larger school.

Consider Enrolling Him in Summer Courses to Start

Why? During summer, classes are typically smaller, and the school's pace seems more laid back. Plus, instructors are typically less busy, so they have more time to spend with individual students.

Check Out Remedial, Developmental, or Preparatory Programs

These transition courses help students ease into campus life. Some—such as study skills courses—are entirely devoted to helping students adjust to college life and "make the grade."

Start Small

Encourage your child to take a reduced course load to begin with. Many youngsters with AD/HD need extra time to do assignments and study for tests, and a full load of courses can seem overwhelming. Plus, you want your child to have ample time to enjoy the nonacademic benefits of college—such as athletics, socializing, and cultural events.

Balance Course Work

Be careful that your child doesn't sign up for too many heavy reading classes all at once (history, biology, literature, psychology, and so forth). His attention span may not stretch that far and he may be doomed to fail.

Help Your Child Brush Up on Independent Living Skills

Before sending your child with AD/HD off to school, get her used to handling such things as grocery shopping, making a budget, balancing a checkbook, paying bills, doing laundry, and cleaning house. The fewer new skills she must learn at school, the less overwhelmed—and more successful—she's likely to be.

Set Up an Appointment with Your Child's Physician to Review His Medication Schedule

The schedule your child followed in high school may not be appropriate for his college or technical-school schedule. Talk to the doctor about your child's new class and homework/study schedule. Sometimes returning to fast-acting medications to cover in-class times and several hours of homework and study sessions each day are sufficient for a child who is inattentive. In other cases, maintaining a long-acting dose with boosters of fast-acting medicine may provide maximum benefits.

Insist that She Continue Her Medication

Many youngsters with AD/HD consider going off to school as an opportunity to "wipe the slate clean." They figure no one knows about them at college, so they can abandon all forms of treatment. Don't let that happen.

Warn Your Child About Stimulant Abuse— and About the Dangers of Mixing Stimulants with Illegal Drugs or Alcohol

Stimulant medication is being abused at increasing rates on college campuses, where students call Ritalin "Vitamin R" or "R-Ball." Some use it for late-night study sessions; others crush up pills and snort them to get high. In fact, when University of Wisconsin researchers recently conducted a formal survey of student Ritalin use, they were shocked at their findings. At least half of the students knew someone who was misusing Ritalin, and about 20 percent had done so themselves.

For this reason, students who have prescriptions for stimulant medications often feel pressured to share them—or their pills may even be stolen from them. Thus, be sure to impress upon your child the need to keep her medication in a safe place. Also, remind her that, since stimulants are a controlled substance, it's not just unsafe to share these drugs with others; it's also illegal.

Encourage Your Child to Get Help When He Needs It

In high school, teachers might automatically have helped your child when he struggled. In college, your child with AD/HD may have to speak up when he needs assistance. Thus, let him practice how he'll explain his disorder to an instructor in simple, clear language. Also, encourage him to consider joining a support group for students with learning disabilities.

Pack Your Child's Suitcase with Plenty of Organizational Tools

These might include packages of sticky notes that can be affixed to books, book bags, alarm clocks, and dorm room mirrors to serve as a reminder of deadlines and things that need to be done. Include organizers, calendars, and agenda books as well as a calculator, pocket spell-checker, and word-processing program with spelling and grammar checkers.

Perhaps tops on your list should be a pocket tape recorder. These are particularly valuable for students who have difficulty writing essays and term papers. What often occurs with children who have AD/HD is that they have a great idea in their head, but they lose their train of thought once they start writing. A pocket tape recorder allows them to tape their thoughts and then transcribe them to paper.

Above all, send your child off to school with a pep talk. After all, children with AD/HD often thrive in college—for a host of reasons. For starters, one-quarter to one-third of youngsters with AD/HD seem to outgrow at least some symptoms by their late teens or early twenties. They may not fully outgrow AD/HD, but many do learn ways to cope with the disorder.

After high school, there is more flexibility, which means they can structure their days around their strengths. If your child tends to focus better in the morning, for example, she can schedule most of her classes at that time.

Finally, while high-school learning tends to be more rigid, college learning calls for more individualized thinking. And this often allows youngsters with AD/HD to use their creativity—and shine!

Preparing Your Child for the Work World

Suppose your child has had his fill of education—at least for now—and prefers getting a job after high-school graduation. If you had higher aspirations for him, don't fret. Taking an entry-level position in business or industry at a young age gives youngsters plenty of opportunities to work their way up the line with promotions over the years. Indeed, in companies that offer good benefits and career ladders, many young people who entered the job market following high school are doing as well as or better than many college graduates. They often retire earlier with better benefits. Not to mention that they are young enough to go back to school or begin another career if they wish.

But will having AD/HD affect your child's ability to succeed in the workplace? Most likely. Fortunately, however, there are strategies parents can use to help make this transition go as smoothly as possible:

Talk to Your Child About What He Wants to Do for a Living

Some children know from the time they are toddlers what they want to be, and they don't veer from that course. A recent sixteen-year-old Olympic gold medal figure skater was video-taped at the age of five talking about winning the Olympic gold medal. On the flip side, some college seniors still don't know what they want to be.

Early career awareness and career planning are assets for helping steer your child on a productive course. Career awareness involves exposing your child to various career opportunities, talking about what a person does in that job, and pointing out people who do different jobs when you are out and about with your child. Career planning takes this process a step further by first matching your child's strengths, weaknesses, and interests with various careers.

And how does having AD/HD figure into this process? An active and fidgety individual would probably not do well as an accountant. But she might shine as a teacher or salesperson, where moving around and dynamism are assets. A child who has struggled with reading throughout school but has an excellent mechanical aptitude has many good options, which should begin with the career/vocational program in high school. Following high school, mechanical aptitudes can be further developed in a vocational technical school or by taking an apprenticeship or a job in industry.

Set Up an Appointment with Your Child's High-School Guidance Counselor

This professional can help with career planning by evaluating your child's strengths and weaknesses and academic performance and by administering career inventories and aptitude tests. The results of these tests can be very valuable in helping your child take that giant step out of your home into a new and promising life.

Don't Rush Your Child out the Door

Entering the workforce requires grooming and maturity, which may be elusive qualities for youngsters with AD/HD. It is not unusual to work several "introduction to work" jobs before entering a career track position. Yet, since these basic jobs rarely pay much more than minimum wage, your child's departure from home may be delayed until he enters a career track position. On the bright side, this extra time offers you an opportunity to reinforce the structure and self-discipline required for job success.

Encourage Him to Be Honest About His Disorder When Applying for Jobs

If a job application asks for information that might interfere with your child's work performance, it's better to be honest up

front about AD/HD. Many workplaces also require drug testing. This means that your child must include on the application
all prescribed medication he is taking so as not to be penalized
on drug-screening tests. You may also need to run interference
for your child, so that his employer will keep you informed of
potential adverse actions if your child is chronically late for
work, shows poor work performance, dresses inappropriately,
and so forth. After all, you want the work experience to be
positive, since it represents your child's future.

Preparing Your Child for the Military

For youngsters who meet the increasingly stringent requirements for enlistment, the military offers some of the best
opportunities available to those who choose not to go to college or technical school. Actually, the structure and discipline
provided by the military can be extremely beneficial for young
adults with AD/HD. Plus, the training, advancement, housing,
pay, socialization, and recreational components make the military an ideal setting for youngsters who have not set their
sights on other career goals.

If your child expresses an interest in joining the military,
here's how you can help.

Sign Him Up for ROTC in High School

Many children begin their premilitary experience in these programs. High-school ROTC offers excellent training for a child
with AD/HD. The uniform that students wear one day each
week can provide positive recognition and boost a child's self-
esteem. What's more, the emphasis on following rules, showing leadership, and maintaining high moral standards may
generalize to other aspects of your child's school and community life.

Talk with Military Recruiters

Like high-school guidance counselors, military recruiters often administer career tests to see if your child and the military would be a good fit. Take note, however, that some branches of the military have limitations on enlistment of individuals who have taken stimulant medication. Generally, a certain number of years must have passed since the prospective enlistee last took medication.

Whether your child dreams of going to college or technical school, getting a job, or joining the military, some time during high school she will make the transition from a pediatrician to a family physician. Having professionals available whom you and your child can trust is important to help resolve problems as your child grows. Other mental health professionals, such as psychologists and counselors, can also help make conflicts, challenges, and barriers resolvable rites of passage in your child's life.

Sharing experiences with other parents who have children with AD/HD at community support meetings can point you in the direction of highly qualified local professionals. In addition, chat rooms on the Internet may provide guidance for specific and unique problems that you are facing. Check the Appendix for reliable Internet sites.

CHAPTER

11

AD/HD IN ADULTHOOD

Three years ago, Jake barely graduated from high school. His parents had always promised him a college education, but Jake had had enough of school. "I was tired of studying so hard and then making all C's and D's," he says. So Jake found a job in construction.

After a year on the job, Jake decided he didn't want to spend the rest of his life building houses. He applied to a small junior college and was accepted. "The classes were small, and students got a lot of personal attention," Jake says, "so I thought if I worked hard I could do well." But with so many social activities going on around him, Jake found he couldn't concentrate on his studies. And by the end of his first semester he was on probation.

The next semester, Jake passed one course but failed two others and was suspended. "I went back home to look for a job," he recalls. "My parents were disappointed in me, and I was disgusted with myself."

Over the next six months, Jake quit one job and was fired from two others. "I felt so restless," he says. "I

couldn't concentrate on anything. Finally, my parents
suggested that I seek professional help, and my mom
made an appointment for me to see a psychologist."

Following testing and an analysis of Jake's school
and family history, the psychologist diagnosed Jake as
having AD/HD. "Neither my parents nor I knew much
about AD/HD," he says. "But as soon as my doctor listed
the symptoms, I knew I'd had it since about second
grade."

Six months ago, at the age of twenty, Jake began tak-
ing stimulant medication. "It's made a tremendous
difference in my life," he says. "I can concentrate at
work. I can relax at home. I feel better about myself
than I have in years."

Jake recently began taking evening classes at a
nearby community college. "Believe it or not, I'm study-
ing psychology." He laughs. "I know it might take me
forever to reach my goal of becoming a psychologist,
but I feel sure I can make it. It's my dream to someday
be able to help children who have AD/HD—so they
don't have to go through the years of hell that I did."

Jake's story is not unusual. AD/HD in adults is a relatively new
phenomenon, yet research clearly suggests that countless
adults had AD/HD as children but were never—and may still
not be—diagnosed. And more often than not, their life stories
sound a lot like Jake's.

Diagnosis in Adulthood

AD/HD in adults is far more difficult to diagnose than it is in
children. In fact, in adults, it's often called "the hidden disorder," despite affecting two to four percent of the adult population. That's because its symptoms aren't so obvious, or they are

attributed to character flaws. For example, someone we think of as extremely absentminded, irresponsible, impulsive, impatient, or restless could very well have AD/HD.

It's not surprising that adults with AD/HD are more likely to have difficulties maintaining social relationships and often have troubled marriages. Many also suffer on the job. They may not follow through on tasks, may be chronically late for work, and often have trouble getting along with colleagues and supervisors.

Adults with AD/HD tend to get bored easily and may move from one unfinished task to another. More often than not, they are major procrastinators and are very disorganized. Many also show poor self-control and can be extremely impulsive— which often makes them risk-takers or substance abusers.

It's not unusual for grown-ups with AD/HD to fidget a lot, get impatient, or be short-tempered while sitting through long meetings or waiting for traffic lights to change from red to green. Many with this disorder are known to wear out their television remote controls. When stressed, adults with AD/HD are typically quick to become anxious, angry, or confused. Finally, few are avid readers, since they can rarely comprehend or remember what they have read.

Clearly, adults with AD/HD face the same kinds of failure and frustration that children with this disorder do. And it is these frequent failures that can perpetuate feelings of poor self-esteem and often lead to unemployment, divorce, and even abuse of tobacco, alcohol, or drugs.

Of course, AD/HD doesn't begin at age twenty, or thirty, or forty. In fact, research reveals that approximately two-thirds of children who had AD/HD continue to have symptoms into adulthood. For this reason, most adults with this disorder need only walk down memory lane to discover patterns that have been there since childhood.

A psychiatrist friend devoted thirty years of his practice to adults with depression and anxiety disorders. As more literature appeared on adult AD/HD, he became more interested in the common histories his patients shared with him about their difficulties in school—not being able to complete work or stay in their seats, having difficulty making friends, underachieving, and rarely meeting their own or anyone else's expectations despite people telling them how bright they were. He began to view his patients' anxiety and depression and their collateral problems on their jobs, in their families, and within themselves as a natural evolution of undiagnosed and untreated AD/HD in childhood. When he began treating their AD/HD as part of their total presenting problems, his patients realized significant positive changes.

Consider this humorous yet sadly accurate account of a day in the life of an adult with AD/HD:

I decide to do the laundry. I start down the hall and notice the newspaper on the table. Okay, I'm going to do the laundry. But first, I'm going to read the newspaper. After that, I notice mail on the table. Okay, I'll just put the newspaper in the recycle stack. But first, I'll look through the pile of mail and see if there are any bills to be paid. Yes. Now where is the checkbook? Oops. There's the empty glass from yesterday on the coffee table. I'm going to look for that checkbook. But first, I need to put the glass in the sink. I head for the kitchen, look out the window, and notice my poor flowers need a drink of water. I put the glass in the sink and there's the remote for the TV on the kitchen counter. What's it doing here? I'll just put it away. But first, I need to water those plants. I head for the door and, aargh! I step on the dog. The dog needs to be fed. Okay, I'll put the remote away and water the plants. But first, I need to feed the dog. End of day: Laundry is not done, newspapers are still on the floor, glass is still in the sink, bills are not paid, checkbook is still lost, and the dog ate the remote control. And, when I try to figure out how come nothing got done today, I'm baffled because I was busy all day!

That Eureka Moment

For many adults, having a child diagnosed with AD/HD is their first clue that they, too, may have this disorder. Jennifer's story is a good example. Recently, Jennifer's ten-year-old daughter, Caitlin, began having problems at school. "She couldn't seem to get organized, and her grades were slipping," says Jennifer. And at home, unless Jennifer sat down with her daughter in the afternoon or early evening, homework would be left untouched. Instead, Caitlin would plant herself in front of the television set or wander around the house.

In school, Caitlin's teachers complained that she often appeared "lost in space." She wasn't focusing on class work and rarely turned in her homework. Finally, Jennifer arranged for her daughter to see a psychologist, who diagnosed Caitlin with AD/HD. And as Jennifer learned more and more about the disorder from various professionals—as well as from books she'd bought and local support meetings she had attended— she began reevaluating her own life.

As a young child, Jennifer had been abused. Although everyone always considered her to be bright, she struggled in school. Still, she managed to make it through high school and shortly after graduation, got married and had two children. Her husband was an alcoholic, however, and the marriage ended in divorce.

As a single mom, Jennifer supported her family by working as an office manager, where she was given many high-level responsibilities. Her supervisors and coworkers frequently commended Jennifer for being so capable and responsible. Nevertheless, she always harbored feelings of self-doubt, was restless, and felt mentally disorganized.

Managing all of these feelings required enormous energy. But Jennifer was always determined to meet others' expectations of her—even if it meant struggling—because she felt it was important to do so for the sake of her children and to keep her job.

Finally, Jennifer made an appointment with a psychiatrist who had recently begun seeing adults with AD/HD. While her daughter, Caitlin, continued to receive treatment for AD/HD, Jennifer was prescribed stimulant medication. The effects were dramatic. "Close friends and associates noticed a difference in me without knowing that I had started taking medication," she reports. "I felt a calmness and clarity of thinking that I had never experienced before. Best of all, I felt a tremendous sense of relief knowing that my constant struggles in life were due to factors over which I had little control!"

There were other benefits as well. Jennifer was able to better understand her daughter's problems and to offer strategies for helping Caitlin improve both in school and at home. In other words, with proper treatment, both Caitlin and her mom appeared to be on the road to a brighter future.

Treatment

Just like children with AD/HD, adults with this disorder benefit most from a multimodal treatment approach. That is, most reductions in symptoms of AD/HD are likely to occur with a combination of medication and other treatment approaches. What's more, these other treatments must be tailored to the very individualized needs of the adult. In other words, dealing with AD/HD in adulthood requires overcoming the cumulative effects of a childhood full of frustration and unfulfilled promise. And this is often quite a different process from treating a child or an adult who has been treated since childhood.

Some adults will need more information on AD/HD and self-monitoring strategies. Others will benefit from parent training to reverse dysfunctional ways of responding to their children. Still others may benefit from counseling regarding their organizational skills, interpersonal relationships, time management, and vocational/career guidance. Some may also need supportive therapy that includes involving the entire family.

Neither can coexisting conditions be ignored. Adults with AD/HD may need counseling, medication, or both to treat depression and anxiety, for example, until these are alleviated by increased feelings of self-control and empowerment.

Finding Help

Due to the complexity, subtlety, and masking of symptoms, there are few professionals in most communities who are comfortable diagnosing AD/HD in adults. Your search for a referral to a qualified professional may begin with your family physician, your child's pediatrician, attending a community AD/HD seminar, or articles in the local newspaper. The most reliable referrals come from trusted professionals or trusted friends.

Try to avoid responding to advertisements or randomly picking a name out of the phone book, however, as credentials and expertise are important when diagnosing and treating this disorder. Your best bet is to find someone knowledgeable about AD/HD and someone you feel comfortable working with as you make your journey to feelings of greater self-worth, control, and success.

12

THE MANY FACES OF AD/HD: A COLLECTION OF CASE STUDIES

This chapter features a number of actual case studies of real children with AD/HD. These case studies show the various ways in which the disorder can be manifested in different children. The notes and comments section that follows each case illustrates the variety of treatments that can be used to help youngsters with AD/HD—as well as their parents and teachers—cope with the disorder.

Chad

Chad, five and a half years old, attends kindergarten at a public elementary school. Because of difficult and disruptive behavior at home, his parents had Chad screened at a mental health hospital to identify possible emotional problems. The screening process, during which a psychologist interviewed Chad and had his parents complete a checklist, revealed that Chad needed additional tests to pinpoint his specific problems.

Chad's parents describe him as a very active and loud child. They say he stays up late at night, has slept with them nightly for many years, and has a bedwetting problem. Chad's father is an alcoholic and there is a great deal of fighting between his parents at home. Chad is an only child who likes to watch cartoons and play outdoors. When he is indoors, his mother describes him as "always into something." Chad also has a mild articulation disorder in which he substitutes the *w* sound for the *r* sound, saying "woom," for example, instead of "room."

Chad had been getting into trouble consistently since the beginning of the school year. Notes from his teacher, describing both his disruptive behavior and the approaches she had used, were a daily occurrence. His teacher has tried time-out, positive reinforcement, one-on-one discussions, restriction of privileges, and other reasonable approaches. Nevertheless, Chad continued to have a difficult time sitting still for activities and completing tasks. At group table activities, Chad was constantly out of his seat, distracted away from the activity, speaking out of turn, misusing materials, and wandering away.

A behavior management strategy was applied at home to structure Chad's bedtime routine. The first step in the plan was designed to make his parents feel more in control of Chad's behavior, as well as to give them some extra time in the evening that was free of direct caregiving responsibilities. Chad was given the choice of sleeping in his own bed with the door open or with it closed. His parents reported that Chad slept in his bed all night by the third night of the program. They were also given suggestions regarding bedwetting: cutting out fluids after 7:00 P.M. and having Chad empty his bladder before going to bed. While his bedwetting decreased, it did not disappear completely.

Chad's parents adopted other behavior management approaches, including use of a contingency approach and time-out. Both reported feeling more competent in being able to use these strategies successfully. However, Chad's behavior did not improve substantially in school or at home. His teacher was very helpful in trying various approaches and keeping a log of Chad's behavior.

His parents shared reports of Chad's response to behavior management at school and at home with his pediatrician. The pediatrician began Chad on a trial of fast-acting Ritalin that Chad took with breakfast and lunch. She also encouraged the continuation of behavior management strategies.

Chad's parents began giving him the medication on the weekend so they could observe changes before sending him to school with medication. They noticed dramatic improvements in his attention and activity level. These changes continued into the school week, except that there appeared to be a regression in his behavior in the late morning, just before his second dose of medication. After a trial of moving the second dose up an hour, it was determined that this would not provide sufficient coverage for the entire school day. Therefore, the morning dose was increased slightly and the noontime dose kept the same for a while. This strategy provided excellent results and allowed Chad to do well academically, behaviorally, and socially in school. Eventually, Chad was changed to Metadate, which worked well through the day and provided the parents with assistance in behavior control at home, as well.

Notes and Comments

When a child shows multiple problems relating to such things as bedtime, mealtimes, interaction with friends, and academics, a plan must be developed to address all these concerns in an organized manner. While medication may be effective in addressing some aspects of the problem, it is not a substitute for sound and consistent behavior management. Nor should it replace other traditional approaches for dealing with such things as bedwetting. Both immediate and long-term success may well depend on more than just dealing with the problems that are most apparent and disruptive to the parents and teachers. Good solutions begin with a realistic evaluation that considers the comprehensive needs of the child within the family, the school, and the community.

Richard

Six and a half years old, Richard is in the first grade at a public school. Last year in kindergarten, Richard was having difficulty getting his work done and paying attention in class. Because he was overweight, some of the other children made fun of him and Richard was unable to make friends. In addition, his teacher would constantly send home notes about Richard's poor behavior. She would also send Richard home with all his incomplete and sloppy papers to complete and redo. Home became Richard's school away from school, and the majority of his afternoons, evenings, and weekends were spent trying to finish his papers. After two months of this, his mother decided to teach Richard at home. She figured that, at the very least, home-schooling might shelter him from the taunting of other students and his very negative teacher.

Soon, however, his mother discovered that Richard had a hard time working for more than fifteen or thirty seconds on a task without becoming distracted and wanting to get up and move around. Academically, Richard did extremely well, but paper-and-pencil tasks and focusing on written and spoken material for long periods of time were difficult for him. His mother tried a number of strategies—brief breaks after short segments of teaching, interspersing passive and active tasks, and using a multisensory approach. Still, Richard's problems persisted.

Richard was tried on Ritalin but showed a significant decrease in appetite and had difficulty falling asleep. Since he was overweight, the decrease in appetite did not pose a risk, but his difficulty getting to sleep was quite severe. After many adjustments in dose, Richard was tried on Adderall. This appeared to provide considerable improvement in his attention with fewer side-effects. For the remainder of the kindergarten year, Richard was taught at home and made excellent progress. He returned to public school at the beginning of the first grade. But his problems were not over.

Despite the fact that his mother took great pains to describe Richard's characteristics from the outset of the first grade, his teacher frequently sent home notes and made Richard redo all his papers when they were sloppy or when the spacing was not perfect. Soon Richard began tearing and shredding his papers or rolling them in a ball and stuffing them in his desk.

Richard never earned Friday treats, which were reserved for children who demonstrated good behavior and work skills throughout the week. Although he talked about wanting to earn treats and was disappointed when he didn't, he was never able to reach that goal. After a few weeks of trying his best to earn a treat, he confided to his parents that he didn't think he could ever do it.

His teacher's notes reported that Richard made noises in the classroom, would get up to sharpen his pencil many times during the day, and had the messiest desk in the class. Richard still managed to make good grades, despite the fact that he was forced to redo his work time and time again. His grades in conduct and handwriting, however, were unsatisfactory.

A Student Support Team meeting was requested. Richard's parents, his teacher, the assistant principal, and a peer teacher attended. His parents, who had two other children at home and were expecting their fourth child in a few weeks, took great pains to describe how they withstood much of Richard's less disruptive behavior. "When we go to church, Richard squirms in his seat and makes a lot of noises, but we have learned to ignore those actions because that's just Richard," his mother reported. "If we got on him for every one of those actions, he wouldn't have a chance to breathe without us pointing out something he was doing wrong. We tried saying things like, 'Richard, sit still and be quiet.' But in less than a minute, he'd be doing the same thing. He just can't help it."

Richard's teacher listened with skepticism. "Well," she said, "we can't have that kind of behavior in the classroom. If I didn't put a stop to it quickly, all of the other children would start behaving that way." The assistant principal pointed out that, since the teacher had not been able to put a stop to Richard's behavior quickly or any other way, perhaps other strategies could be identified to redirect Richard's inappropriate behavior without continually sending negative messages to him. It was suggested, for example, that Richard be given an opportunity to assist other children in math and reading once he had completed his own seatwork. Considering that he was a bright child and at the top of his class academically, maybe he needed the social interaction and would feel good about having the opportunity to help other children. The group concluded that this might be a way to motivate Richard to complete his work quickly and to avoid other disruptive behavior. Richard's medication level was increased and the school counselor taught him techniques to help him gain better self-control. These strategies appeared to have a positive effect. However, his teacher did little to change her approach in the classroom and had Richard's performance not improved as a result of these other strategies, a trial period in another classroom would have been recommended.

Notes and Comments

There is little to gain by developing an adversarial relationship between parent and school. On the other hand, parents have a right to stand up for the best interests of their child when they feel that he is not benefiting from the educational environment. They should have some confidence that educators are interested in the welfare of their child, and this should be reflected in the efforts of the school to exhaust all strategies to help the child adjust and succeed in that setting. When things are not working, the parents should ask the question, "What can we all do?" And after having an opportunity to try out a different strategy, they should ask, "Did it work?"

Failure to follow through on suggested strategies may result in frustration at both ends. Parents may feel that the school is not doing its share to carry out what was proposed. School personnel may also be frustrated that the parents are not following through on commitments they have made. At times such as this, especially when the child is not experiencing improvement, it is often beneficial to adopt the *pleasant militant* approach we described earlier or to seek the help of an outside person who can view the needs of the child in a more objective way. Finding such a person is the parents' responsibility. The person may be another parent, a psychologist, a counselor, or some other individual familiar with AD/HD and school matters.

Alan

Alan is fourteen years old. From his infancy on, Alan's parents have described their son as a difficult child. Compared to his brother and sister, as an infant he was fussier, slept fewer hours, and ate less. His parents remember Alan often waking up crying during the night and being extremely difficult to console.

During the toddler years, when Alan could not play outside, he would mope around the house. He also had a difficult time staying clean and dry during the day until he was nearly four years old and he continued to wet his bed almost nightly until he was eight.

As Alan grew older, he had a difficult time keeping friends. When he was in second grade, his parents, concerned about his poor growth and continual reports from his teachers about his inattention and inability to complete work, took their son to the nearest university medical center for an evaluation. After a thorough medical evaluation, plus a review of behavior checklists by his parents and a narrative report from his teacher, Alan was prescribed hormone therapy for a growth disorder, along with Ritalin. After a period of dose adjustments of Ritalin, the supervising physician changed his prescription to Adderall. The growth hormone therapy was discontinued after three years, but Alan continued to take Adderall with inconsistent results.

Now in the eighth grade, Alan has had a history of increasing problems over the years. His progress is now being followed by a private pediatrician rather than the medical center. His parents say Alan has started fires, broken into a neighbor's house, stolen a bicycle, and done poorly in school. These behavioral episodes have been sporadic, but his poor academic performance has been consistent over the years.

Reports from current teachers indicate that Alan behaves well in school and has no apparent problems paying attention and completing his work. However, they say that Alan does not appear very motivated and often will not hand in his homework or take the time to answer questions completely.

A Daily Report Card was initiated with rapid and positive results. With performance in class tied to recreational privileges at home, Alan's grades improved dramatically after just a few weeks. He also admitted to being pleased with the change and attributed it to the use of the Daily Report Card.

Following this success, the parents and Alan canceled or failed to appear for many of their scheduled appointments with their psychologist. Six weeks after his last contact with Alan and during the spring vacation, the psychologist received a call from Alan's mother. Her son and some of his friends had broken into a home in the neighborhood and stolen money and other goods. Alan's mother was frantic. She and her husband had been extremely proud of their son for the improvements he had recently shown in school. His mother was now distraught over what steps to take in dealing with the current problem.

Notes and Comments

Alan's case reflects a number of very critical points about children with AD/HD. First, AD/HD may coexist with many other problems and disorders. In addition, the persistent impulsiveness and frustration that is a part of AD/HD may contribute to other problems such as conduct disorders and delinquent-type behavior. Finally, parents often feel that, when the attention problem and the most significant current problem (in this case, poor academic performance), appear to be under control, contact with the professional is no longer needed.

Alan is small in stature, which was the reason growth hormone therapy was prescribed, and which contributed to his feelings of inadequacy. Many children who are small for their age look to a peer group for acceptance. And, unfortunately, the maxim "Birds of a feather flock together" often pertains to children who have problems. Associating with other difficult children, together with a tendency toward impulsiveness, was a combustible combination that kept Alan in trouble.

It is not surprising that the episode of breaking into someone's house occurred during vacation time. Alan's academic performance improved when increased structure was added. During school days, he had a very regimented routine that helped him to be more successful. However, during vacation, the structure was gone. His parents let down their guard, and consequently, Alan reverted to greater impulsivity. In addition, Alan did not take his medication, which is consistent with drug holidays recommended by many physicians for children who are on chronic medication.

Alan's pediatrician indicated to his parents that he would no longer write refills for medication unless Alan's progress was being monitored by a psychologist or counselor. If this stipulation was met, he wanted Alan to take the medication daily rather than just on school days. The parents, shaken by their son's recent setback, agreed to their pediatrician's stipulation.

In spite of the financial burden of medical care, Alan's parents felt reassured that they would now have somewhere to turn to avoid or to better deal with crises. In fact, Alan continued to make excellent progress and his parents have had many opportunities to be proud of each of their three children.

Jamie

Jamie is a three-year-old whose parents have experienced severe marital problems. Jamie's mother recently filed for divorce because of her husband's physical and emotional absence from the home and because of his unwillingness to spend much time with their son. Jamie's mother was troubled and frustrated by her son's behavior. She had recently taken him to a department store, and the manager asked her not to return because of Jamie's destructive and disruptive behavior. She revealed that, no matter where they go, Jamie misbehaves. He runs away from her at the mall, wants to touch everything at the grocery store, is constantly interrupting her when she is on the phone or visiting with friends, and always touches things at home that he's been told are off-limits.

Jamie's mother is very health-conscious and has been systematic about keeping her son away from artificial food additives, chocolate, sweets, and other dietary items that might contribute to his high activity level and impulsiveness. This approach has not improved Jamie's behavior. She has also used time-out and has awarded or taken away privileges, depending on Jamie's behavior.

Because of the severity and consistency of Jamie's poor behavior, a trial on stimulant medication was recommended together with behavior management approaches, described in a publication that the pediatrician gave the mother. Jamie was started on a low dose of generic Ritalin (methylphenidate hydrochloride). After three days, his mother saw no change in her son's behavior. The morning dose was increased slightly, resulting in only a mild change in behavior. Before abandoning this strategy altogether, Jamie was tried on brand-name Ritalin. The first day his mother reported that Jamie appeared wide-eyed and lethargic. However, on the second and subsequent days, she saw a dramatic improvement in his performance. She had several meetings set up with lawyers to discuss her pending divorce, and Jamie sat quietly at the lawyer's office reading and writing while she had her meetings. She had never experienced this pleasant occurrence with Jamie before. No side-effects from the medication were noted.

Notes and Comments

Behavioral intervention always should be tried before using medication. Moreover, while use of medication is less desirable with young children than with older children, it must be considered when the behavior is severe enough to interfere with normal family life and the child's preacademic and social success.

When children who show Jamie's characteristics come from a dysfunctional family, it can be difficult to sort out an environmental problem from an organic one. A systematic management strategy can help shed light on the causes for the given behavior. Often environmental and organic problems combine to create the difficult behavior.

Finally, some children respond differently to the generic forms of AD/HD medication. Thus, it's usually a good idea to begin children on the brand name and consider changing to the less expensive generic form, when available, after the success of the medication and the correct dose have been established.

Mary

Thirteen-year-old Mary is in the seventh grade at a public school. She has been in the same school where her mother taught. She was recently referred to a psychologist for assistance because of poor grades and a lack of motivation.

Both of Mary's parents are professionals. She also has two older sisters, both of whom do well in school. Mary plays the flute in the school band, plays soccer, and is a very creative and inventive child. Nevertheless, she has shown inconsistency in her school work—not doing homework assignments and projects on time, forgetting her responsibilities, losing things often, and exhibiting a general pattern of disorganization.

A review of Mary's past school work indicates average to above-average scores on standardized tests, such as the Iowa Test of Basic Skills and the Cognitive Abilities Test. She received mostly grades of B and C at the private school she attended but has made mostly C's, D's, and an occasional F since transferring to public school. Mary's poor grades frustrate her parents tremendously, since they have worked very hard to provide her with assistance and support throughout her school career. It appears that the demands of the upper grades are the main factor in Mary's decreasing grades, both on her report card and on tests. Her parents have tried many behavioral strategies and incentives at home. Over the years her teachers have also tried many interventions without consistent success. As a result of Mary's problems in school, she is also beginning to show increasing evidence of poor self-esteem, talking about feeling stupid and not being able to do anything right.

Mary's psychologist recommended a trial on stimulant medication to Mary's physician. She was begun on a dose of 20 mg of Metadate CD in the morning. Since Mary was not thrilled about the idea of taking medication, a contract was set up whereby she agreed to try it over a three-week period; at the end of that time, she would have the right to choose not to use it any longer if she thought it was not helping. Together with the medication, Mary started using a marker board in her room to maintain lists of things she needed to remember and tasks she had to complete. She also began carrying a pad of "sticky" notes along with her to record items she needed to remember. She would attach these notes to the top of her books.

As a result of these interventions, Mary's productivity and attitude improved noticeably. She expressed an ability to concentrate better and understand more of what she was reading. She complained periodically of headaches. Her mother says that Mary has always complained of one ailment or another, but that the complaints rarely persist. This pattern of persistent complaints subsided, however, following the introduction of Metadate. Periodic headaches were treated with traditional remedies.

Notes and Comments

AD/HD is particularly difficult to identify in adolescents. Because inconsistent behavior, changing priorities, and adjustment to physical changes are typical of youngsters at this age, many adolescents display characteristics that may lead others to suspect that they have AD/HD. In such cases, it is extremely important to review a child's educational history for indications that the characteristics were present *before* adolescence. This information may come from comments that teachers made on report cards in the early grades, from discrepancies between a child's standardized test scores and school grades, from reports by parents about the child's difficulty getting homework done and completing school work, and from other sources. Even with this documentation, the child should currently meet the criteria specified for AD/HD relating to inattentiveness, impulsiveness, and distractibility.

Adolescents often feel invincible and have a difficult time admitting that they have problems. Consequently, many will resist the idea of taking medication and almost certainly will object to taking it at school. In such cases, the use of long-acting medication is desirable. This avoids the need for a child to deal with the perceived embarrassment of having to take medicine at school and having to explain why she is taking it.

Finally, medication by itself is rarely sufficient treatment. This is especially true for children who have experienced many years of frustration and disorganization. It is necessary to help these youngsters learn techniques to become better organized and more efficient. Parents who have characteristics of AD/HD have probably learned some tricks along the way to help them be more successful. Sharing these strategies with their children can be helpful. Likewise, strategies that are recommended for children with AD/HD may also be beneficial to adults. In fact, an entire household can be made more efficient by strategically placing marker boards throughout the house. This helps all family members keep track of one another and of tasks that need to be completed.

Thomas

Twelve-year-old Thomas lives with his grandparents. His parents were divorced several years ago. They were substance abusers who moved around often, and Thomas attended many schools before his grandparents enrolled him in a private school last year. He is currently in the seventh grade.

Teachers describe Thomas as a very likable and athletic child. Nevertheless, they indicate that he is aggressive, impulsive, and has a hard time getting along with other children as well as getting his work done. At home, Thomas is mildly defiant with his grandparents but has some chores around the house that he does regularly without having to be told many times. His grades have been marginal throughout his academic life, although his standardized test scores have always been in the high-average to above-average range. Apparently, the great importance placed on these tests by the school and family—or the way these particular tests are administered—has allowed Thomas to compensate and excel on these types of tests.

Thomas sees his mother occasionally and his father a little more often. None of these visits occurs more than once or twice a month, however. Thomas has spent most of his life living with his grandparents, who have tended to pamper him. He has no desire to live with either of his parents.

Thomas was certainly underachieving and showed many symptoms of AD/HD. The first step in treatment was to initiate a Daily Report Card to get a better idea of his day-to-day performance in school. When this strategy was explained to Thomas, he seemed eager to try it. An evaluation of his Daily Report Card at the end of the first week was extremely positive. Thomas seemed to appreciate the structure that this approach imposed on him and enjoyed the positive feedback that he got from his grandparents daily.

After two weeks, when it was suggested that the Daily Report Card be discontinued for a short time, Thomas balked and insisted on continuing the procedure. Thomas's grades and attitude have improved consistently over time and problems at home have decreased, although there have still been a few episodes of defiance and rebellion, which is not unusual for a child his age. His grandparents now feel more capable of being consistent with Thomas, since much of the pressure to motivate him to improve his school work has been taken off them.

Notes and Comments

Just as in Mary's case, a careful analysis of many factors is needed to untangle and understand Thomas's problems. It is clear that a nurturing and loving environment alone does not guarantee success. Children need structure and consistency; when these are absent, youngsters typically "ask" for these qualities in various ways. In Thomas's case, what appears to be a very complex and significant problem may have a fairly simple solution. Clear rules with clear consequences were what Thomas needed to bring his behavior and academic performance more in line.

Arthur

When Arthur was in the fourth grade, he did well on tests but rarely finished his seatwork. His teacher would send home all his unfinished papers; thus, in addition to the thirty to forty minutes of homework that she expected all her students to do each night, she also expected Arthur to complete his unfinished papers. Unfortunately, forty minutes' worth of homework for most fourth-graders took Arthur two to three hours. With his unfinished class work added to the homework load, all of Arthur's time—and his parents'—was spent on homework. Life was miserable for him and for the whole family.

Arthur's parents met with his teacher on a number of occasions to discuss their child's problems, but the teacher said it was Arthur's responsibility to get his work done and that "maybe his parents shouldn't baby him quite so much." This infuriated and frustrated Arthur's parents, particularly since they had tried every strategy they knew to get their child working on his own. They used incentives. They tried spanking him. They sent him to his room. They took away his privileges. Nothing had worked.

Finally, Arthur's parents were referred to a professional who recommended that they request a Student Support Team (SST) meeting. The parents recruited an advocate to accompany them to a meeting with Arthur's teacher, the school administrator, and a peer teacher. During this meeting, the school representatives expressed little sympathy for Arthur's plight. They warned his parents about how much more difficult things would be when Arthur got into middle school and how nobody would coddle him in the advanced grades.

The parents' advocate countered with a request that several steps, consistent with the recommended structure of SST meetings, be taken at that time:

- That Arthur's teacher and his parents describe the problem.
- That the teacher discuss her suggestions for how to resolve the problem and that the parents describe strategies they had used at home.
- That the group agree that all logical approaches had been used to resolve the problem and that a modification of expectations for Arthur be made, given the fact that his grades were good and he appeared to know the work but had difficulty demonstrating his knowledge in traditional ways.
- That the SST meet again in one month to review Arthur's response to the modifications.

Notes and Comments

It is rare to find school professionals these days who have not heard of Attention Deficit/Hyperactivity Disorder. Unfortunately, there still are a few and an even larger number who know about the disorder but are not willing to listen to the concerns of parents of a child with AD/HD or to make accommodations to meet the needs of these children and their families. This is what happened with Arthur and his parents in their attempt to get the school to respond to their concerns. In the end, however, the parents' advocate was able to negotiate a solution.

The advocate suggested—and Arthur's teacher finally agreed—that Arthur work no more than one and a half hours on homework and school work on any night. At the end of that time, work would be put away and unfinished class work would be sent back to the teacher. In addition—and, again, with great reluctance—the teacher consented to try other approaches in the classroom to help Arthur get his class work done. She also agreed not to send home more than one class assignment each day.

As the year proceeded, as well as in subsequent years, Arthur continued to make good grades. Home life became considerably less frustrating and more enjoyable for the whole family.

At a recent two-year follow-up, Arthur was still having to spend a good bit of time doing his homework but appeared to be motivated and was earning good grades. Home life also continued to be less stressful than it had been in the fourth grade.

It is unfortunate when parents must seek outside help to pressure the schools to fulfill their responsibilities. Indeed, many school personnel are very committed to children and do everything within their means to assist. Sometimes this is not enough for children whose problems are severe or for whom other nonschool professional intervention is needed. Moreover, sometimes the problem is so unusual that outside resources are needed to provide guidance. But AD/HD is now recognized as a common problem and schools must join with parents—rather than take sides against them—to do the right thing for the child. And for children who do not respond to the school strategies recommended by the SST, testing by the school psychologist may be appropriate with consideration for special education placement or modification under Section 504 (see page 119). The parents must also consider talking with their pediatrician when modifications have been consistently unsuccessful in improving the child's performance.

Matt

Matt is a five-year-old who was adopted at the age of two. He was in foster care from the age of three months until soon after his second birthday. In his original environment, he suffered extreme deprivation. The foster home in which he lived for nearly two years was also a neglectful environment.

Currently, Matt lives with his adoptive mother and his older sister and brother, both of whom were adopted from other families. The adoptive parents are divorced and the children live with their mother. Matt is characterized as a combative child who is defiant toward authority and unpredictable in his behavior. His teacher says Matt has "fits" in school, where he is likely to throw a chair, knock everything off his desk, or attack another child when he is corrected or told to do something he doesn't want to do.

Matt is in a kindergarten class in a private school and shows problems staying on task and learning new songs and poems. He enjoys going to school but is unpredictable in his behavior once there. He shows language delays, particularly in the use of pronouns (for example, "Me want some"), and has had speech articulation problems involving sound substitutions.

When Matt came into the office for an evaluation, he wrote holding his pencil with a full hand grasp. When the evaluator tried correcting Matt's pencil grip, the child began fighting and tugging at the evaluator. "You're not taking it from me," he said. He called the evaluator stupid and kicked him.

During formal testing, Matt was cooperative but moved around a lot. On standardized tests, he scored high in spatial and math skills, but low in language and memory skills. Matt clearly met the criteria for AD/HD, although his history and current behavior suggested a more deeply rooted emotional disorder.

Given Matt's background of neglect, as well as his current behavioral and social problems, the evaluator weighed two options: an intensive psychiatric workup or a short-term trial on stimulant medication before referral for additional services. The evaluator decided to recommend to Matt's physician a preliminary trial on medication.

Matt was started on a low dose of Ritalin. Reports from his teacher were instantaneous and positive. The change in Matt's behavior at home was also dramatic. His behavior was more consistent, he was beginning and completing his work more efficiently, and he was interacting in a more friendly way with other children. Matt and his mother continue to receive counseling, and Matt appears to be a much happier and productive child, showing only intermittent episodes of the type of combativeness that had earlier been a regular part of his repertoire.

Notes and Comments

There are no easy and definitive answers to the problems of some children with AD/HD. This is particularly true when the child's current behavior is complicated by a very significant past history. In such instances, critical and delicate decisions must be made to find the quickest solution to a problem without doing any additional harm.

Behavior intervention programs alone to help children with severe emotional problems have yielded inconsistent results and often require long periods of time before progress is seen. Consequently, the decision to try Matt on Ritalin was made with the understanding that the trial would be monitored closely and was extremely unlikely to do him any harm. The benefits, however, might be significant.

Nevertheless, given the extensiveness of the problems, it is important that Matt and his other family members be involved in regular counseling with the goal of helping Matt and his family members deal with current and future demands.

Sara

Sara is six years old. Since she was old enough to walk and talk, Sara had been having severe temper tantrums, didn't sleep well, was a picky eater, and argued constantly with everyone. The intensity of her problems increased as Sara entered new social situations and reached dramatic proportions when she began kindergarten. All behavior management strategies appeared ineffective with Sara. Home life was chaotic—not only for Sara but for her parents and her three older siblings.

When Sara entered kindergarten, she was put on Adderall. The medication was effective for a brief period of time, yet even at high doses it did not allow her to maintain enough self-control to function well in the classroom or at home. In addition, her appetite and sleep patterns remained poor.

After several months of adjusting doses and schedules, Sara began to exhibit eye-scrunching and uncontrollable sniffing. Since these tics, it was felt, were the result of her medication, Sara was changed to Ritalin. On this medication, she began rolling her eyes and clearing her throat a great deal, and she continued sniffing. And while her behavior improved briefly at each dose level, improvement was never maintained.

Over several months, many meetings were held at school to change Sara's workload, to improve communication between the school and home, and to discuss other ways to evaluate Sara's progress. Finally, it was decided that Sara would be taken off all medication for a period of time to see how she would respond. The tics decreased but did not disappear, and her behavior and productivity remained extremely inconsistent.

Sara was referred to a neurologist, who diagnosed Tourette's syndrome and began Sara on clonodine. The tics decreased substantially and there was some improvement in her behavior. The dose of medication was eventually increased to the point where Sara was given a transdermal patch to wear. Unfortunately, she was not able to tolerate the adhesive from the patch and had to resume taking the medication orally. Stimulant medication was reintroduced.

Classroom and home modifications continued with modest improvement in work and behavior. Treatment then focused on reintegrating Sara into the family unit so that there was more enjoyment among family members, as well as less emphasis on Sara's problems and more emphasis on her accomplishments.

Notes and Comments

Many parents who have children with AD/HD will relate to Sara's story. Family life is never totally free from stress and anxiety. Some families experience continual bouts with modifying behavioral approaches and medications, observing changes, and modifying and adjusting still more.

Sara represents one of approximately 15 percent of children with AD/HD who are resistant to most interventions. Discovering what will help Sara be more consistently successful requires a delicate combination of factors. First, someone must be available who can provide suggestions and help monitor intervention—a type of case manager. Second, Sara's parents and teachers must be willing and able to apply behavioral interventions and to modify these fairly consistently based on their observations and other objective and subjective evaluations of progress. Finally, Sara must have medical services available that will consider the use of less traditional medical interventions when traditional ones are ineffective.

The side-effects that Sara experienced from the various medications serve as a reminder that few medications are totally free of possible negative side-effects. When those side-effects are not life-threatening, the physician may closely weigh the benefits of the medication against the frequency and intensity of the side-effects when deciding whether to continue with that medication. In all cases, whenever a new medication is prescribed or a dose is changed, parents must be especially vigilant for both undesirable physical changes in the child's behavior (such as rashes and eye-blinking) and complaints of discomfort.

When flexibility, consistent intervention, and good medical care are present, even children who appear to be resistant to treatment will show some benefits. Above all, good communication with the children is a necessity. That way, she will have a good understanding of both her limitations and the efforts she can make to improve her performance—and she can take pride in her accomplishments.

APPENDIX

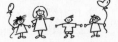

Resources for Parents

ADDitude magazine. (P.O. Box 2687, Houston, TX 77252, 1-800-856-2032.)

Anderson, W, Chitwood, S, and Hayden, D (1990). *Negotiating the special education maze: A guide for parents and teachers.* Bethesda: Woodbine House.

Attention! magazine. (www.chadd.org or 1-301-306-7070.)

Barkley, RA (2000). *Taking charge of ADHD* (revised). New York: Guilford Press.

Dendy, CAZ (1995). *Teenagers with ADD: A parent's guide.* Bethesda: Woodbine House.

Hallowell, EM, and Ratey, J (1995). *Driven to distraction.* New York: Pantheon.

Lynn, GT (1996). *Survival strategies for parenting your ADD child.* Grass Valley, Calif.: Underwood Books.

Nadeau, KG, Littman, E, and Quinn, PO (2001). *Understanding girls with AD/HD.* Silver Spring, Md.: Advantage Books.

Power, TJ, Karustis, JL, and Habbouishe, DF (2001). *Homework success for children with ADHD: A family school intervention program.* New York: Guilford Press.

Quinn, PO (2001). *ADD and the college student* (revised). Washington, D.C.: Magination Press.

Taymans, JM, and West, LL (2000). *Unlocking potential: College and other choices for people with LD and AD/HD.* Bethesda: Woodbine House.

Wachtel, AC (1998). *The attention deficit answer book.* New York: Plume (Penguin) Press.

WEBSITES

www.chadd.org	Children and Adults with Attention Deficit/Hyperactivity Disorders
www.add.org	The National Attention Deficit Disorder Association
www.tsa-usa.org	Tourette's syndrome Association
www.adaa.org	Anxiety Disorders Association of America
www.interdys.org	International Dyslexia Association
www.ncld.org	National Center for Learning Disabilities
www.cabf.org	Children and Adolescents Bipolar Foundation
www.adhd.ucla.edu	Reports on genetic research projects at UCLA
www.cec.sped.org	Council for Exceptional Children
www.fape.org	Information for families on IDEA
www.addwarehouse. com	Comprehensive source of materials on AD/HD
www.ldonline.org	A variety of information on learning disabilities
www.jan.wvu.edu	Information on job recommendations and work for individuals with disabilities
www.nichcy.org	National Information Clearinghouse on Children and Youth with Disabilities
www.protectionand advocacy.com	National network of disability rights agencies
www.ffcmh.org	Federation of Families for Children's Mental Health

www.nmha.org	National Mental Health Association
www.psych.org	American Psychiatric Association
www.apa.org	American Psychological Association
www.aap.org	American Academy of Pediatrics
www.intelihealth.com	Harvard University's Consumer Health Information Site
www.nimh.nih.gov	National Institute of Mental Health
www.nlm.nih.gov	National Library of Medicine
www.aacap.org	American Academy of Child and Adolescent Psychiatry
www.aboutourkids.org	Comprehensive site of the NYU Child Study Center, including current material on AD/HD
www.addvance.com	A resource for women and girls with AD/HD

RESOURCES FOR CHILDREN

Bramer, JS (1996). *Succeeding in college with attention deficit disorders.* Plantation, Fla.: Specialty Press.

Carpenter, P, and Ford, M (2000). *Sparky's excellent misadventures: My A.D.D. journal.* Washington, D.C.: Magination Press.

Crist, J (1996). *ADHD: A teenager's guide.* King of Prussia, Pa.: Center for Applied Psychology.

Galvin, M (2001). *Otto learns about his medicine: A story about medication for children with ADHD* (3d ed.) Washington, D.C.: Magination Press.

Gantos, J (2002). *Joey Pigza loses control.* New York: Farrar.

Gantos, J (2000). *Joey Pigza swallowed the key.* New York: Farrar.

Janover, C (1997). *Zipper, the kid with AD/HD.* Bethesda: Woodbine House.

Moss, DM (1989). *Shelley, the hyperactive turtle.* Bethesda: Woodbine House.

Nadeau, KG, and Dixon, EB (1997). *Learning to slow down and pay attention: A book for kids about ADD.* Washington, D.C.: Magination Press.

Quinn, PO, and Stern, JM (2001). *Putting on the brakes: Young people's guide to understanding attention deficit hyperactivity disorder* (revised). Washington, D.C.: Magination Press.

Quinn, PO, and Stern, JM (2000). *The best of brakes: An activity book for kids with ADD.* Washington, D.C.: Magination Press.

BIBLIOGRAPHY

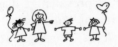

American Psychiatric Association (1994). *Diagnostic and statistical manual of mental disorders* (4th ed.). Washington, D.C.: author.

Barkley, RA (1998). *Attention deficit hyperactivity disorders: A handbook for diagnosis and treatment.* New York: Guilford Press.

Biederman, J, Wilens, T, et al. (1999). Pharmacotherapy of attention deficit/hyperactivity disorder reduces risk for substance use disorder. *Pediatrics,* 104:2.

Brown, TE (2000). *Attention-deficit disorders and comorbidities in children, adolescents, and adults.* Washington, D.C.: American Psychiatric Publishing Group.

Castellanos, FX (2001). Neural substrates of attention-deficit hyperactivity disorder. *Advances in Neurology,* 85: 197–206.

Castellanos, FX (1999). Stimulants and tic disorders: From dogma to data. *Archives of General Psychiatry,* 56(4): 337–38.

Ch.A.D.D. (2000). The ChADD Information and Resource Guide. Landover, Md.

Chan, E (2002). The role of complementary and alternative medicine in attention-deficit hyperactivity disorder. *Journal of Developmental and Behavioral Pediatrics,* 23 (1 suppl): 537–45.

Chan, E (2002). The role of complementary and alternative medicine in attention-deficit hyperactivity disorder. *Journal of Developmental and Behavioral Pediatrics,* 23 (suppl): s37–45.

Chervin, RD, et al. (2002). Inattention, hyperactivity, and symptoms of sleep-disordered breathing. *Pediatrics,* 104(3), 449–56.

Conner, DF (2002). Preschool attention deficit hyperactivity disorder: A review of prevalence, diagnosis, neurobiology, and stimulant treatment. *Journal of Developmental and Behavioral Pediatrics,* 23 (1 suppl): S1–9.

Doyle, AE, and Faraone, SV (2002). Familial links between attention deficit hyperactivity disorder, conduct disorder, and bipolar disorder. *Current Psychiatry Reports,* 4:146–52.

Evans, SW, Pelham, WE, Smith, BH, Bukstein, D, Gnagy, EM, Greiner, AR, Altenderfer, L, and Baron-Myak, C (2001). Dose-response effects of methylphenidate on ecologically valid measures of academic performance and classroom behavior in adolescents with ADHD. *Experimental and Clinical Psychopharmacology,* 9:163–75.

Fisher, SE, Francks, C, et al. (2002). A genomewide scan for loci involved in attention-deficit/hyperactivity disorder. *American Journal of Human Genetics,* 28 (epub).

Gershon, J (2002). A meta-analytic review of gender differences in ADHD. *Journal of Attention Disorders,* 5:143–54.

Giedd, JN, Blumenthal, J, Molloy, E, and Castellanos, FX (2001). Brain imaging of attention deficit/hyperactivity disorder. *Annals of the New York Academy of Sciences,* 931:33–49.

Hirsch, GS (2001). Anxiety disorders and AD/HD. *Attention,* 8(3): 34–39.

Kurlan, R (2002). Methylphenidate to treat ADHD is not contraindicated in children with tics. *Movement Disorders,* 17(1):5–6.

Mick, E, Biederman, J, Faraone, SV, Sayer, J, and Kleinman, S (2002). Case-control study of attention-deficit hyperactivity disorder and maternal smoking, alcohol use, and drug use during pregnancy. *Journal of the American Academy of Child and Adolescent Psychiatry,* 41:378–85.

Mick, E, Biederman, J, Prince, J, Fischer, MJ, and Faraone, SV (2002). Impact of low birth weight on attention-deficit hyperactivity disorder. *Journal of Developmental and Behavioral Pediatrics,* 23:16–22.

MTA Cooperative Group (1999). A 14-month randomized clinical trial of treatment strategies for attention deficit hyperactivity disorder: *Archives of General Psychiatry,* 56: 12.

Nass, R, and Bressman, S (2002). Attention deficit hyperactivity disorder and Tourette's syndrome: What's the best treatment? *Neurology,* 58, 513–14.

New York University School of Medicine (2002). Treating attention-deficit/hyperactivity disorder (AD/HD) in school settings. *Child Study Center Letter,* 6(5):1–6.

Papolos, DE, and Papolos, J (2001). Bipolar disorder & AD/HD: A diagnostic conundrum. *Attention,* 8(3): 28–33.

Pliszka, SR, Carlson, CL, and Swanson, JM (2001). *ADHD with comorbid disorders.* New York: Guilford Press.

Quinn, PO, M.D. Top ten things I wish students with ADHD knew about their medications. *ALERT: The Official Newsletter of the Association on Higher Education and Disability.* April 1998, Volume 22 (2).

Robin, AL (2000). *ADHD in adolescents: Diagnosis and treatment.* New York: Guilford Press.

Sergeant JA, Geurts, H, and Oosterlaan, J (2002). How specific is a deficit of executive functioning for attention-deficit/hyperactivity disorder? *Behavior and Brain Research,* 130:3–28.

Sonuga-Barke, EJ, Daley, D, Thompson, M, Laver-Bradbury, C, and Weeks, A (2001). Parent-based therapies for preschool attention-deficit/hyperactivity disorder: A randomized, controlled trial with a community sample. *Journal of the American Academy of Child and Adolescent Psychiatry,* 40:402–8.

Swamson, JM, and Volkow, N (2002). Pharmacokinetic and pharmacodynamic properties of stimulants: Implications for the design of new treatments for ADHD. *Behavior and Brain Research,* 130:73–78.

Tannock, R, and Martinussen, R (2001). Reconceptualizing ADHD. *Educational Leadership,* 59(3): 1–8.

Taymans, JM, West, LL, and Sullivan, M (2000). *Unlocking potential: College and other choices for people with LD and AD/HD.* Bethesda: Woodbine House.

Voigt, RG, Llorente, AM, Jensen, CL, Fraley, JK, Beretta, MC, and Heird, WC (2001). A randomized, double-blind, placebo-controlled trial of docosahexaenoic acid supplementation in children with attention-deficit/hyperactivity disorder. *Journal of Pediatrics,* 139:189–96.

Weiss, M, Hechtman, LT, et al. (1999). *ADHD in adulthood: A guide to current theory, diagnosis, and treatment.* Baltimore: Johns Hopkins University Press.

Wilens, T (2001). Effects of AD/HD medication on future substance abuse. *Attention* 8(3): 40–43.

Wilens, TE, Biederman, J, et al. (2002). Psychiatric comorbidity and functioning in clinically referred preschool children and school-age youths with ADHD. *Journal of the American Academy of Child and Adolescent Psychiatry,* 41(3): 262–68.

Williams, G III. Hyperactivity hype. *Parenting,* September 2000, pp. 120–29.

INDEX